FOR THOSE WHO LIVE AND BREATHE

A Manual for Patients with Emphysema and Chronic Bronchitis

Second Edition, Second Printing

By

THOMAS L. PETTY, M.D.

Associate Professor of Medicine
Head, Division of Pulmonary Diseases
University of Colorado School of Medicine
Denver, Colorado

and

LOUISE M. NETT, R.N., A.R.I.T.

Coordinator, Respiratory Care Unit
University of Colorado School of Medicine
Denver, Colorado

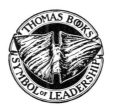

CHARLES C THOMAS · PUBLISHER
Springfield · Illinois · U.S.A.

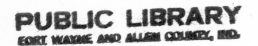
Published and Distributed Throughout the World by
CHARLES C THOMAS • PUBLISHER
BANNERSTONE HOUSE
301-327 East Lawrence Avenue, Springfield, Illinois, U.S.A.

© *1967 and 1972, by* CHARLES C THOMAS • PUBLISHER
ISBN 0-398-02380-8
Library of Congress Catalog Card Number 78-184610

First Edition, First Printing, 1967
First Edition, Second Printing, 1969
Second Edition, 1972
Second Edition, Second Printing, 1975

With THOMAS BOOKS *careful attention is given to all details of manufacturing and design. It is the Publisher's desire to present books that are satisfactory as to their physical qualities and artistic possibilities and appropriate for their particular use.* THOMAS BOOKS *will be true to those laws of quality that assure a good name and good will.*

Printed in the United States of America
N-1

Preface to Second Edition

THE PURPOSE OF THE first edition was to explain emphysema and chronic bronchitis as well as the management of these two important diseases to the patient and his family and friends. We allowed our enthusiasm for the care and management of these problems to permeate the book and hoped that what we offered would provide realistic comfort to some of the fifteen millions of Americans with these problems.

Over four years later, following further research, evaluation of treatment methods and a study of the natural course of emphysema and chronic bronchitis, we remain extremely enthusiastic and pleased over prospects for care and prevention.

We feel the acquisition of new knowledge through research and the development of improved technology are sufficient reasons to write this second edition. Our reevaluation of the total situation has caused us to completely reorganize this book and to make additional emphasis on early identification, treatment of reversible features and to make an all-out appeal against smoking and air pollution, two factors which unquestionably cause damage to the lung.

Much of what we wrote in the last chapter, "The Outlook and the Future," we now find in the daily practice of medicine. Additional factors such as hereditary weaknesses in the lungs' defenses against injury have become known.

Today we face the future with new hopes that an enlightened public will place greater efforts on prevention and early identification of disease and that research now in progress will provide even better methods of care, treatment and rehabilitation.

THOMAS L. PETTY, M.D.
LOUISE M. NETT, R.N., A.R.I.T.

v

Preface to First Edition

THIS BOOK IS WRITTEN for the two million patients known to be suffering from emphysema and chronic bronchitis today, as well as for their friends and families who need to know the nature and treatment of these two important diseases.

It has been estimated that as many as 10 per cent of middle-aged and elderly American males suffer from emphysema and chronic bronchitis today. These two conditions are more prevalent than tuberculosis and lung cancer combined. The great impact of these diseases is underlined by the fact that eighty million dollars is paid by Social Security annually for chronic lung disability, second only to heart disease. For this reason, both federal and private agencies are now studying the feasibility of developing screening and prevention programs, as well as intensive care and rehabilitation programs for patients with emphysema and chronic bronchitis. A major purpose of this book is to explain and stress the true rehabilitation potential for patients with these two lung diseases.

We began to write this book because of frustration concerning the air of hopelessness and despair that patients and many physicians have concerning the treatment and care of these associated diseases. This book is also written because of our concern that existing knowledge is often not used today to treat and prevent these diseases.

This book is also born of enthusiasm. We now know that emphysema and chronic bronchitis are diseases for which effective treatment and rehabilitation are possible. We know that many patients improve through medical treatment and can learn to live comfortable productive lives once again.

This book is written in plain language. It is designed simply to explain and describe what is known about emphysema and chronic bronchitis today. We also provide detailed advice on rehabilitation and adapting one's life to the burden of these two diseases.

We are convinced that patients with emphysema and chronic bronchitis must understand their diseases and the objectives of therapy in order that they may participate in the care that doctors, nurses, and physical therapists are offering. Replacing fear with knowledge opens many avenues of self-help for the patient with chronic lung disease.

The first chapters are devoted to medical facts and clear-cut descriptions concerning these diseases. A final glossary gives definitions of the medical terms as they apply in the text. These terms are italicized when first used throughout the twelve chapters of the book.

Most of the book is designed to describe current medical, surgical and rehabilitation programs for emphysema and chronic bronchitis. Chapters on medication, use of nebulizers, oxygen therapy, use of breathing machines, and bronchial hygiene will enhance each patient's knowledge of his own individual care and what is expected from treatment. We know that the enlightened patient can best cope with his disease.

Important portions of the book are those chapters concerning day-to-day living and suggestions concerning methods of adjusting to emphysema and chronic bronchitis.

The last chapter, "Outlook Today and the Future," is based upon our own research now taking place in our Respiratory Care Laboratory as well as that from a number of other university medical centers.

This book must be dedicated to our patients. These individuals living today have been a constant source of inspiration, new ideas, and hope for the others with emphysema and chronic bronchitis. These patients with tremendous courage have clamored for guide lines on how to live and breathe despite, often times, serious disease. They tell us more patients should be taught about what is known and understood concerning the care and rehabilitation of patients with emphysema and chronic bronchitis — thus we present this book to them.

We hope that the readers who are patients with these diseases will gain insight into their own care as they read this book. We have added a number of anecdotes, some of which are personal and some of which have been given us by patients, in order to underline and emphasize some of the predicaments patients or their physicians and nurses encounter in the care of emphysema and chronic bronchitis. We hope further that readers will find humor in bits of verse scattered throughout the book. They were given to us by our colleagues and patients. Humor is our policy and our book would not reflect the personality of patients or ourselves without it.

We would like to acknowledge with appreciation the secretarial work of Mrs. Martha Melton, Miss Jean Finlayson, Miss Lynn Salters and Mrs. Mary Ann Hammond.

THOMAS L. PETTY, M.D.
LOUISE M. NETT, R.N.
1967

Note: Figures 2, 6, 7, 10, 11, 21, 22, 23, and 24 are reprinted from *Medical Times* with permission.

Figure 13 is reprinted from *Intensive and Rehabilitative Respiratory Care,* Lea and Febiger with permission.

Acknowledgments

T HE AUTHORS WISH to acknowledge our present colleagues involved in the field of respiratory care: Virginia Carpenter, Martha Conway, Georgia Foss, Ellen Musick, Ellene Sander, Elizabeth Schatz, G. Wayne Silvers, Alan Suzuki, Martha Tyler, and Patty Way.

Contents

FOR THOSE WHO LIVE
AND BREATHE

Chapter I

The Lungs

THE LUNGS ARE MAGNIFICENT ORGANS. The two lungs continuously fill and empty bringing new oxygen to the blood stream and removing carbon dioxide, the waste product of body function (*metabolism*). To accomplish normal oxygenation and carbon dioxide removal, the lungs are filled and emptied with approximately 12,000 quarts of air each day.

It should be stressed that respiration is fundamental to all forms of higher animal life. Even the single cell ameba exists by virtue of *oxygen transport* and carbon dioxide removal through the cell membrane.

The human organism, the most complex of all life, needs a very efficient system of oxygenation and carbon dioxide removal. Our lungs are so structured as to be able to handle the fantastic amount of air necessary to support life. To compare, the body can function without food for several days and without water one to two days, but cannot be without oxygen for more than a matter of minutes.

The lungs comprise multiple smaller units which include five lobes (3 on the right and 2 on the left) (Fig. 1). The lungs are made up of a series of branching tubes (Fig. 2), and a delicate membrane for gas exchange (Fig. 3). The branching tubes are the conducting airways and it is the purpose of these structures to transport fresh air to the gas exchange membrane.

The *trachea* is the main airway; it branches into a *bronchus* for each lung. The trachea and bronchi have a certain rigidity by virtue of cartilage which strengthens these larger tubes. From this point onward, twenty successive orders of branching occur until the conducting airways end in a series of blind sacs called *"alveoli."* These sacs comprise the alveolar membrane. The membrane allows the passage of oxygen into the blood stream and the outward passage of carbon dioxide, the product of the body's metabolism (Fig. 4) to exit from the blood. Each alveolus or alveolar

3

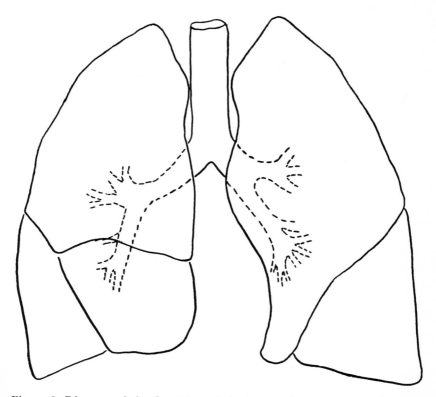

Figure 1. Diagram of the five lobes of the lung and the corresponding conducting airways. According to medical orientation, the right lung (three lobes) is on the reader's left and the left lung (two lobes) is on the reader's right.

wall contains numerous elastic fibers which allow these structures to expand on *inspiration* and contract on *expiration* individually and together as the lung inflates and deflates. In spite of their delicacy, the alveoli are durable and do not wear out throughout the millions of breaths which stretch alveoli in the normal course of breathing. Age itself does not damage the lungs. The size of the alveolar membrane is astonishing. Whereas each alveolus is so small that ten to fifteen equal the size of a pinhead, if all the individual tiny sacs were rolled out to form a flat surface, the area of the lung membrane would measure about 400 square yards.

This is approximately the size of a tennis court, and is about a fifth the size of a football field. All of the conducting air tubes and alveoli are intermeshed in an *elastic superstructure* which allows the lungs to inflate on inspiration and to recoil on expiration. The lung is encased within a thin sac, the *pleura*, which is really a sac within a sac. The pleural surfaces glide upon each other in inspiration and in expiration. The outer layer of the pleura lines the chest cage or *thorax*.

One might compare the exquisite packaging of the lung within the chest with a parachute and its container. A parachute can be

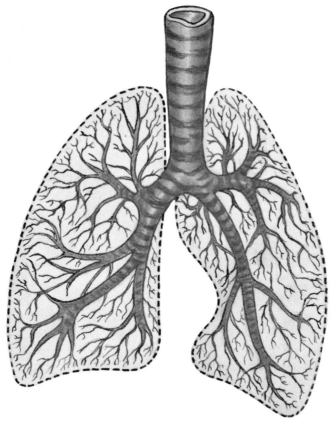

Figure 2. Conducting airways of the lungs. The main airway or trachea (windpipe) divides into a main bronchus for each lung. These further divide by twenty generations of branching until some 50,000 small airways result.

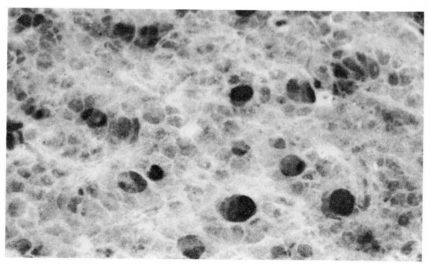

Figure 3. The alveolar gas exchange membrane is a delicate lace-like structure with thousands of small bubbles (alveoli) lining the ends of the conducting airways (alveolar ducts). This provides a maximum surface area for the exchange of oxygen and carbon dioxide.

rolled upon itself until it fills a package which is strapped to the back. This parachute now occupies a space somewhat smaller than the chest. When unfurled, the same parachute would cover one's back yard or even the greater part of the tennis court we are using for comparison.

The power for breathing or for filling and emptying the lungs comes from the chest muscles. These are the diaphragm (the large piston-like muscle in the chest and abdomen) and the muscles of the thorax (Fig. 5). A coordinated act of chest expansion obliges the passive lungs to follow suit and expand in conformity with the chest. This act of inspiration in essence "sucks" the air into the lungs. Expiration is normally performed with no effort. A relaxation of the muscles of inspiration allows the chest to become smaller and the lungs recoil because of their own elasticity. This process is like inflating a balloon by forced air, and then allowing the balloon to empty again by itself because of its own elasticity.

In the act of normal respiration, the thorax (chest), conduct-

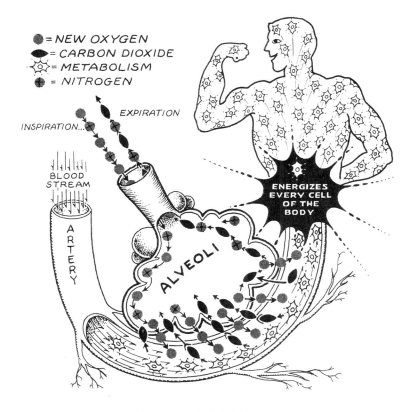

● = NEW OXYGEN
◆ = CARBON DIOXIDE
⚬ = METABOLISM
◉ = NITROGEN

EXPIRATION

INSPIRATION...

BLOOD STREAM

ARTERY

ALVEOLI

ENERGIZES
EVERY CELL
OF THE
BODY

METABOLISM

Figure 4. The artist concept of ventilation and oxygen transport depicted by new oxygen entering the blood stream and carbon dioxide leaving the blood stream entering the alveoli to be expelled. Since oxygen provides the fuel for metabolism, it indeed energizes every cell of the body for aerobic metabolism to support life.

ing airways, alveoli, and elastic structure function together in concert like an orchestra. Normal breathing is almost effortless so that the lungs fill and empty with ease.

This complex process of breathing is controlled by the original computer system, *the respiratory center* of the brain located in the *medulla*. This coordinating center receives all messages concerning the need for more or less breathing and reacts by controlling the lungs and thorax accordingly (Fig. 6).

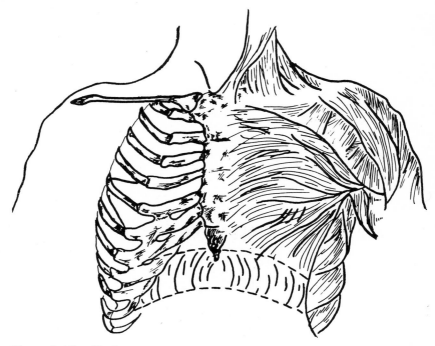

Figure 5. The diaphragm represented by dotted line of the lower part of the figure is a piston-like curved muscle which is elevated on expiration and depressed on inspiration to draw more air into the lungs. This figure depicts the musculature of the thorax on the reader's right and the unexposed ribs to which the muscles of respiration are attached on the reader's left.

The heart pumps blood through a fine *capillary* network into the lungs; the capillaries line the walls of each alveolus. The reason for this is that the main function of the lung, as we understand it, is the exchange of oxygen and carbon dioxide between the outside air and the circulating blood.* Thus, there must be an intimate association between the capillaries which carry the circulating blood from the larger vessels and the alveolar walls which allow the passage and exchange of gases. During the course of twenty-four hours, the heart will pump nearly 6,000 quarts of blood through the lungs. So, with the gale of air entering and leaving the lungs in inspiration and expiration in close contact with a veritable flood of blood being pumped through the lungs

*The lung may have other functions in controlling chemical events of the body.

continuously, it becomes clear that the lungs are very active organs indeed!

Our life is totally dependent upon adequate lung function. To prove this to ourselves, we need only to try to hold our breath for more than a minute or two. A tremendous sense of *air hunger* is

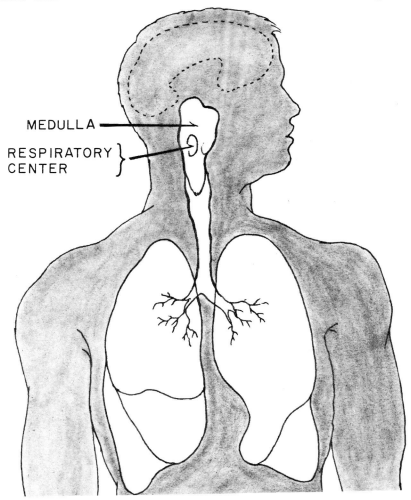

MEDULLA

RESPIRATORY }
CENTER }

Figure 6. Diagram of the respiratory center and its nervous connection to the lungs and thorax. The respiratory center is a computer-like station which receives messages concerning the needs for respiration and controls the muscles of respiration (diaphragm and chest musculature).

the result. Our brain becomes irreparably damaged if blood is inadequately oxygenated to the point that vital brain cells die. Some trained athletes (e.g., swimmers and deep sea divers) can hold their breath for approximately five minutes, during which time life is supported in the tissues by the extraction of nearly all the oxygen from the circulating blood. After four or five minutes, the will to hold one's breath is absolutely overcome by the need to breathe. This personal suffocation experiment is not advised for patients but it tells scientists something of the distress of patients who are forced to fight to breathe each day for existence.

The following is a personal anecdote on breathlessness from Dr. Petty: "I was recently climbing up a steep hill after fishing a small stream. My job was simply to work upward through some tall timber and climb nearly a mile to the car. At 10,000 feet I was short of breath with nearly every step, but all I had to do was climb more slowly and my breath returned. I had achieved my second wind. I thought then that most of my patients are always in 'tall timber' but they can't stop. On a later trip, after exercising each day by walking stairs at work instead of using the elevator and generally exercising more, a similar mile was much more easily performed and shortness of breath did not occur." Later chapters will show the importance of breathing training so that patients can get out of the 'tall timbers' of breathing difficulty. Chapter VIII on physical reconditioning discusses the phenomenon of the "second wind" and how this can be utilized in an exercise program for patients.

In emphysema and chronic bronchitis, in which the airways are obstructed, the work of bringing air in and out of the lungs is great and the patients experience some or much of the distress of "too little air."

The lungs are protected by a variety of mechanisms designed to prevent irritation and damage. Most normal people breathe through the nose. The nose has many functions. It warms or cools the air before it enters the lungs. The nose is a filter and removes *bacteria* and *irritants* before they can enter and damage the lungs. The nose also *humidifies* the air so that it is not excessively dry on entering the lungs.

The conducting air passages of the lungs contain *mucous*

glands, which normally produce a small amount of mucus each day. This is swept upward toward the mouth continuously by small hair-like structure called *cilia* (Fig. 7). The cilia beat rhythmically together in unison so as to sweep the mucus forward toward the mouth and thus cleanse the lungs of inhaled irritants and also to protect the lungs against noxious invaders. The cilia and flowing mucus blanket together are the custodians of the airways. Smoking can paralyze the cilia and thus remove one of our most important guardians of the lung. Cigarette smoke may actually damage the lungs because it leaves the lungs defenseless. On cessation of smoking, however, ciliary activity may recuperate and once again perform the normal function of airway cleansing. This recovery process may take several months following the cessation of smoking.

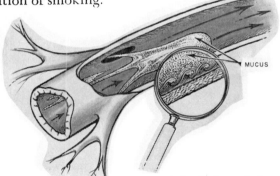

MUCUS

Figure 7. The cilia or hair-like structures of the lining of the airways beat rhythmically in a coordinated fashion to propel a blob of mucus toward the upper airways and mouth for expectoration.

The alveolar walls contain another defense mechanism. Numerous scavenger cells *(macrophages)* are contained in the alveoli. These have the ability to ingest or engulf particles or bacteria and later to float this cargo through the *lymphatic channels* and ultimately to jettison their load into *lymph glands.* The alveolar macrophages are important in combating the dangerous particles which get into the lungs and which are deposited on alveolar walls.

If one ever has the opportunity to view animal or human lungs, one is impressed with the very delicate structure and the elasticity with the pink color of normal lungs. One would see a tremendous contrast in the damaged lungs of emphysema or bronchitis lungs. These lungs would be blackened and full of holes like swiss cheese. This *black pigment* has not been identified, but it probably results, at least partly, from disease. It is also partially related to cigarette smoking.

How Physicians Evaluate the Lungs

Although many patients with both emphysema and chronic bronchitis see physicians frequently, perhaps they do not always understand what the physician is trying to find out in his history-taking and examinations. It is important to know from the history the level of activity which may be performed in comfort by the patient. The number of colds occurring in the chest is recorded and the details of drug therapy reviewed (Chapter V). Since *bronchial hygiene* is of tremendous importance (Chapter VI) the details of this form of therapy are carefully scrutinized. These historical facts help the physician toward any necessary changes in the therapeutic regimen.

On initial evaluation, the physician needs to know how the illness began. The onset is mostly cough in the case of chronic bronchitis and unexplained shortness of breath in emphysema with cough coming on later in this type of illness. By noting the speed of progress of disease the physician can predict something of the future. For example, if the patient's symptoms have leveled off and really are no different this year than two years ago, a slow progress of disease or perhaps no progress is expected. By contrast if an inexorable deterioration is occurring, this is a warning sign that everything possible must be done now to stop the dangerous progress of the disease. Physicians will review the family history of disease, since current evidence indicates a *genetic* component in some family groups. Patterns of colds will help indicate the need for antibiotic therapy. Inquiries concerning digestive function, urinary function, and general muscular strength help allow the physician to size up the patient before his therapeutic efforts begin.

On examination, the physician notes the patient's color. A peculiar blue color may indicate inadequate oxygenation, but it may simply point to the fact that excessive blood is present in conjunction with slightly low oxygen. The physician will note the breathing pattern and the presence or absence of discoordinated inefficient labored breathing. As the physician thumps the chest he notes the hollow sound of the overdistended thorax. By far the most important sign that alerts the physician's attention are the production of so-called *breath sounds*. Breath sounds are made by the entry and exit of air through the conducting airways. In emphysema and chronic bronchitis the breath sounds are decreased because there is obstruction to air flow and thus the sounds point to situations where therapy may help. If a high pitched whistling noise of *wheeze* is heard, this may indicate muscular spasms of the conducting airways and indicate the use of *broncho-dilator therapy* (Chapter V). Bubbling sounds indicate excessive mucus accumulation in the airways and demand a better bronchial hygiene program (Chapter VI). Examination of the heart and the electrocardiogram may determine any excessive sign of strain which may indicate the need for cardiac drugs. The examination of the extremities may show swelling which represents salt and water retention. This often occurs in *heart failure* which frequently accompanies severe *chronic obstructive lung disease.*

X-rays are of tremendous value in identifying new episodes of *pneumonia,* but they are not of great value in estimating the patient's ability to breathe and the degree of disability or the amount of emphysema and or chronic bronchitis. The x-ray picture is somewhat different in emphysema than in chronic bronchitis and there is some value in diagnosis by x-ray.

The electrocardiogram helps indicate strain on the heart. The electrocardiogram is frequently and routinely performed during initial or periodic evaluation in both emphysema and chronic bronchitis. The request of this test by the physician does not necessarily imply that something is amiss with the heart.

Blood counts are frequently done to determine a build-up of *red blood cells* which occurs when low oxygen stimulates the bone marrow to produce excessive blood. Occasionally, this build-up is much too excessive; then therapeutic bleeding (*phlebotomy*) is needed. An elevated *white cell count* may indicate infection.

Sputum examinations help tell the physician what organism is causing a flare-up of bronchitis or pneumonia. Sputum tests are often obtained in the face of a new infection. However, the most common organisms causing flare-ups of bronchitis and pneumonia are well known, and many physicians, quite rightly, institute *antibiotic* therapy without knowledge of the exact organism.

A variety of tests indicate the degree of damage to the lung caused by disease. These are so-called lung function or pulmonary function tests. The most commonly used tests measure the ability to move air in and out of the lungs. This is usually performed by having a patient breathe into a device similar to a canisterer *(spiro-meter)* with the result of breathing recorded. It is now possible to conveniently measure the blood oxygen and carbon dioxide by modern methods, and most hospitals can perform these tests rapidly. Other more sophisticated tests are occasionally performed in order to pinpoint exactly where the problem with oxygenation or carbon dioxide removal exists. Still other tests deal with the work of breathing in the study of patients with chronic bronchitis and emphysema.

Exercise pulmonary function tests are performed often with the patient walking on a treadmill (endless belt) or exercising on a stationary bicycle, or simply stair-stepping. The importance of exercise tests is to study the patient's ability to breathe during activity, the time when patients have most of their symptoms.

In summary, the lungs are complex organs comprising branching tubes which end with the alveolar membrane. Elastic fibers, mucous glands and a circulatory system for the transport of the oxygenated blood away from the lungs and the carbon dioxide laden blood to the lungs are essential for normal lung function and life. The next two chapters show how the lungs may become damaged in emphysema and chronic bronchitis.

Chapter II

What Is Emphysema?

T HE DICTIONARY DEFINITION of emphysema is unsatisfactory. Early Greek physicians coined the term; it literally means "blown up" and "full of air." The Greeks originally used this term to refer to abdominal distension and abdominal gas. The term is quite appropriate, however, for in emphysema the lungs are truly blown up and full of gas — stale air.

The underlying problem in emphysema is destruction of alveolar walls. As described in Chapter I, the alveoli make up the gas-exchange membrane; this is where oxygen is absorbed into the blood and carbon dioxide removed. Recent research has shown that small holes called *fenestrations* begin to form in the alveolar membrane, and these holes enlarge and break into one another forming large tears and eventual rupture of alveoli. This occurs probably long before patients have symptoms of emphysema. When sufficient destruction occurs, the membrane of the lungs becomes full of holes, much like a swiss cheese, with loss of functioning membrane surface. It is easy to understand how loss of alveolar walls leads to loss of surface area of the lungs. If we considered a house with its numerous partitions and wanted to know how much paint it would take to paint all of the walls, we would have to measure the surface area of all the individual walls within the home, that is, both inner and outer wall partitions. If we took all of the partitions out of the house, the overall size would remain the same but the amount of paint necessary to paint only the outer walls would be very much less. We can liken this analogy to how departitioning of alveolar walls leads to less available surface area for gas exchange. At this point, the transport of oxygen and carbon dioxide removal is impaired.

Figure 8 shows the cut section of a normal lung on the left compared to a destroyed emphysematous lung on the right. Figure 9 shows a magnified view of the normal alveolar membrane on the

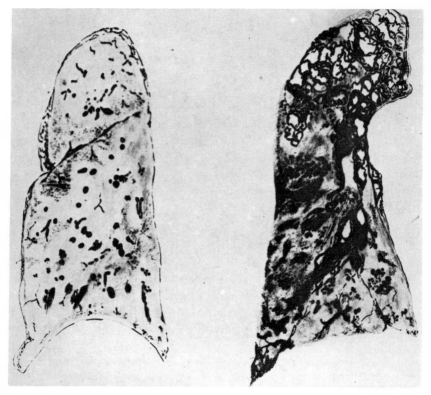

Figure 8. The cut section of a normal lung on the left is compared to the destroyed lung of emphysema on the right (note blackened pigment).

left, described on page 7 (Fig. 4), compared to the blackened, destroyed lung of emphysema on the right.

The lung in emphysema, now riddled with holes, also fails to allow for normal filling and emptying. The elasticity of the lung is lost and one may consider, for comparison, an overstretched balloon. As it loses its stretch it becomes flabby, a distended bag and all of the air put in will not come out. Something else happens. Normally the conducting airways (Chapter I) are held open, partly by the elasticity of surrounding stretchy fibers, something like guy wires. These fibers also lose their elasticity, like a worn-out rubber band, and eventually break. Thus, the lung's outward pull is lost and the airways can collapse like a reed on expiration and stale air is trapped. Figure 10 demonstrates the spring-like

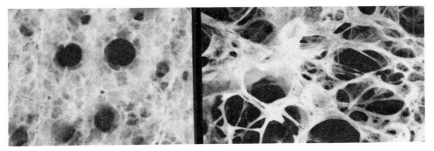

Figure 9. A magnified view of the normal (on left) compared with the destructible process of emphysema leading to residual holes and loss of normal architecture in emphysema (right).

attachments to the conducting airways. Fewer attachments are found in emphysema. Figure 11 shows the collapse of the conducting airways in emphysema compared to normals due largely to loss of the elastic pull of the conducting wall attachments in emphysema patients.

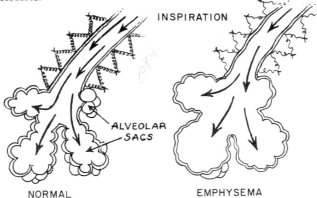

Figure 10. A diagram of the spring-like attachments of the conducting airways. These are lost and reduced in elasticity in emphysematous lungs, but the act of inspiration still allows the air to enter the lungs.

Possibly to compensate for lost elasticity, the lungs of emphysema tend to overexpand in order to become larger and thus to stretch further to regain some elastic pull. This is why patients with emphysema sometimes are said to be "barrel-chested" (Fig. 12) because their lungs and chest are rounded and overexpanded as the process of emphysema develops.

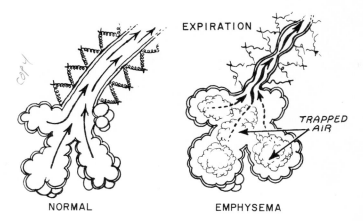

Figure 11. This shows collapsing of conducting airways on expiration in emphysema compared to the normal lungs where patency of the airway is maintained. This is due at least in part to loss of the elastic pull of the conducting wall attachments in emphysema patients (normal on left and emphysema on right).

The cardinal symptom of emphysema is shortness of breath while exercising. Shortness of breath has many other causes, of course, but emphysema is one of the most common. Doctors call shortness of breath *dyspnea*. This occurs at first on severe exercise but as the disease becomes progressive, dyspnea may also be present in varying degrees at rest. The reason the patient is short of breath is that he has to work exceptionally hard to move air in and out of the lungs. It is difficult to move air into the lungs because the lungs are already overexpanded and full of old air. Tremendous effort is needed to force air out of the lungs because the airways collapse and narrow on expiration. In emphysema, exhaling is like blowing through a flabby straw. This process can be overcome in part with breathing training discussed in Chapter VIII.

Another cardinal symptom of emphysema is cough. Coughing may even be the earliest symptom of disease. The term "just a cigarette cough" should alert the physician to future problems. A cigarette cough, a "hacking cough," or a morning cough is not normal. Since so many people smoke and cough, the public has come to accept cough as a normal fact of life. Cough is not normal. Some patients deny they ever cough, but in close questioning or

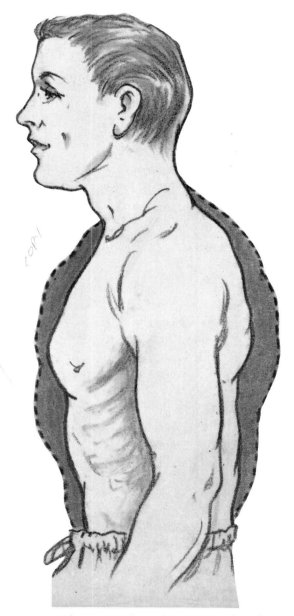

Figure 12. The normal chest configuration compared to the emphysema configuration (shaded area as shown). The emphysema patient tends to overexpand his lungs to try to exert additional pull on the conducting airways.

confrontation or on a separate interview with the spouse, a definite history of cough can often be obtained.

For example, we often count the number of times a patient coughs during the taking of a history. It seems incredible that a patient may literally cough dozens of times in front of the doctor or nurse, but deny he ever coughs. He may even say "I don't ever" (he coughs in the middle of the sentence) "cough." When we say, "What was that?" He says, "I cleared my throat." "It's sinus trouble." "It is a tickle in my throat." Or he may say, "it is only a cigarette cough."

The wife may report that she has retreated to separate bedrooms because "He coughs his head off all night and it keeps me awake."

The reason for cough is that some degree of irritation of the airways is present. Lungs that are damaged by emphysema frequently fall victim to deep chest infections and some degree of constant irritation is often present, both from colds and from smoking. It should be stressed that a closely related disease, chronic bronchitis, frequently coexists with emphysema and, as a matter of fact, in America the two diseases, emphysema and chronic bronchitis, are often lumped together with the term "emphysema" encompassing both groups. Europeans have often used the term "chronic bronchitis" to refer to both diseases. In truth, most patients with emphysema have some degree of chronic bronchitis and most patients with chronic bronchitis have some degree of emphysema.

Another prominent symptom of emphysema is wheeze. This is not usually as dramatic as the wheeze of asthma, but is present in varying degrees among many patients. Wheeze is a whistling noise made on expiration and probably occurs as a result of air whistling through collapsing airways which contain some secretions from associated chronic bronchitis or from a simple irritation.

Why is emphysema harmful? First, patients become worn out by excessive work of breathing. Second, oxygen (Chapters I and IX) is essential to the function of all cells of the body and all tissues are damaged by low oxygen. This leads to wasting of muscle, strain on the heart, indigestion, poor appetite, and mental symptoms. Beyond this burden, the build up of poisonous carbon dioxide occurs late in the course of the disease and as one patient put it, "every organ in the body takes the rap."

The cause of emphysema is not known. Evidence points to an inflammation of the alveolar walls as a factor in destruction, but what actually causes the inflammation is not known with certainty. Current research indicates that the irritating effects of tobacco smoke, air pollution and repeated chest infections cause damage to the lungs leading to the destructive process that results in emphysema. This is why we stress the importance of early treatment of chest infection, the cessation of smoking and the daily removal of secretions in patients with this problem.

It may be that emphysema has many causes. This disease was first noticed and described by Laennec, a brilliant young French physician, who out of his boyish embarrassment from futile examination of buxom females, became the inventor of the *stethoscope*. He first described emphysema in 1819 and at that time smoking was not common, but neither was emphysema.

The disease cannot be found in preserved human mummies of ancient history. Egyptian mummies have been found to have tuberculosis, but no emphysema. Emphysema may have a hereditary component because several members of one family may have the disease.* We recently saw a family in which there were four male farmers with emphysema; three smoked heavily, but one smoked very little.

Some races have very little or no emphysema. We have seen few of Negro heritage or Spanish heritage with the disease. Today, emphysema is not as common in females as in males. We hasten to add that almost all females with emphysema are smokers, but since smoking is a much more recent habit among females, the incidence of disease remains comparatively low, but it is rapidly increasing, paralleling the cigarette habit.

Emphysema may occasionally affect the young and we have cared for a man who died at age twenty-nine. He had smoked for only eight years and previously had been a Marine athlete. Even doctors and nurses are not protected, because these valued friends and colleagues continue to smoke.

*Recently a factor indicative of a high risk of emphysema has been identified in the blood.

Why don't animals get emphysema? Actually, a rare strain of mice occasionally do and so do a few rabbits, but this is unusual. We have even tried to produce emphysema in animals and have failed. So, we must assume that this is a disease of humans.

Later chapters deal with the treatment of emphysema, but we would like to stress at this early stage in our book, that in spite of the many problems found in emphysema patients and with the gaps in our knowledge, we do have effective treatment for both emphysema and chronic bronchitis today.

Chapter III

What Is Chronic Bronchitis?

CHRONIC BRONCHITIS IS A TERM which has been present in the medical literature for many years, but it has also been a waste basket designation applied to anyone with a long-standing cough, "bronchial trouble," or so-called *catarrh* (a term used by Laennec in 1819). Chronic bronchitis has lacked a strict definition — it has been a term waiting to be applied to a disease.

Chronic bronchitis is *inflammation* of the conducting airways. Microscopic studies of these airways reveal a thickening of the lining of the airways and presence of increased secretions as well as inflammation. This inflammatory swelling is what finally interferes with air flow in and out of the lungs because the swollen passages compromise the air space (Fig. 13). We could compare the swollen airways with rusty pipes that eventually become obstructed or plugged.

Patients notice cough particularly in the morning with production of mucus which may or may not contain some color. Often the morning cough is considered a "cigarette cough" or a "hackers

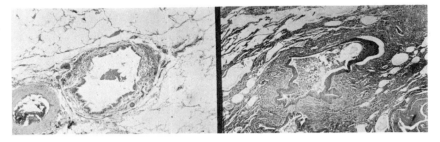

Figure 13. Conducting airway (left) in center of section with only a small amount of mucous in the center conducting airway. Notice normal artery accompanying normal airway. Surrounding lung attachments are seen. Plugged airway (right) with surrounding inflammation. Combination of mucous plugging and inflammation interferes with the conducting space (lumen).

cough" and it is believed to be normal. Since the American public has so completely accepted smoking, even telltale evidence of disease (coughing) is quickly set aside as being insignificant. Patients with chronic bronchitis cough every day for many months or years. Headcolds frequently settle in the chest and cough is then increased. Sputum production is also increased with colds.

When airway narrowing from the swollen glands of bronchitis becomes severe, patients again have to labor to breathe air through the *resistance* of the narrowed tubes. Thus, as in emphysema, shortness of breath occurs. At this point the patient may consult his doctor. Unfortunately, the progression of chronic cough and sputum ultimately leading to narrowing of the airways may take place insidiously and occupy years of time in development. By the time the patient becomes worried because of shortness of breath, extensive inflammation may be present and thus therapy more difficult.

We stress, at this point, that all shortness of breath does not indicate lung disease. Patients may be overweight and out of condition and thus suffer from labored breathing. Current evidence indicates that the irritation and inflammation leading to chronic bronchitis may be caused by four major factors: smoking, infection, *air pollution,* and *allergy.* Smoking is probably the most important factor in the development of chronic bronchitis. A complete review of the hazards of smoking in relation to emphysema and bronchitis is recorded in Chapter IV. Infection also causes inflammation of the lungs, and repeated colds that settle in the chest as well as episodes of bronchitis and pneumonia participate in the inflammatory swelling of the airways. It is likely that air pollution also contributes.

Air pollution is a combination of many active ingredients — products of combustion. Auto exhaust gives forth hydrocarbons and the effects of sunlight on hydrocarbons produces a toxic, irritating gas called ozone. Ozone in high concentration paralyzes the cilia, the main cleansing mechanism of the lung. The importance of lung cleansing was explained in Chapter I. It should be stressed that smoking is the most potent inhibitor of lung cilia (Chapter IV). Air pollution from industry contains many other irritants, all of which can damage the lungs and cause or aggravate chronic bronchitis.

Allergic reactions in the airways, similar to asthmatic reactions, may cause swelling similar to the nasal swelling of hayfever in the conducting passages of the lungs. A combination of chronic bronchitis with allergy is sometimes called asthmatic bronchitis because in this situation both inflammation and allergic swelling are present. Patients with asthmatic bronchitis may have a wheeze as a predominant symptom accompanying a troublesome cough.

It is stressed that the cessation of smoking, the avoidance of air pollution, and the prompt and effective treatment of infection or allergy may halt the course of chronic bronchitis and indeed certain studies suggest that the inflammatory swelling may regress and heal if irritation and inflammation can be avoided or effectively treated. The details of treating and preventing chronic bronchitis are found in the following chapters.

We repeat that patients should not accept morning cough as normal. They should not accept a cigarette cough as part of daily life, and when these symptoms are present, they should immediately take stock of the situation and consult their personal physician. We stress the importance of establishing the diagnosis of chronic bronchitis because the bronchial inflammatory element is what we can treat most effectively.

Some patients, at times, become dramatically better on therapy. All patients are different and one cannot compare his own case with that of his neighbor. We recall an eastern industrialist who came for treatment of "severe emphysema." He was unable to work and had forsaken the normal routine of daily activities. He had generally lost interest in life. Actually, we found that his most important symptom was cough and expectoration and thus we knew that although he had some emphysema, a large part of his problem was his chronic bronchitis or bronchial irritation. After cessation of smoking and after breathing training (details in later chapters), he gradually became free of secretions, able to breathe, able to exercise, interested in life, and returned to work, played golf, and vacationed in Europe.

We saw him a year later for a flare-up in his disease. At that time we learned that he was smoking again. He was definitely worse but had not completely deteriorated. After the same treatments and again after stopping smoking, he made a similar recovery and once again returned to work. We believe the important message here is that effective treatment can reverse the bronchitic element and return the patient to useful life.

Chapter IV

Smoking and Air Pollution

SINCE SMOKING IS A MAJOR if not the most important single factor in the development of chronic bronchitis and emphysema, the entire book might be devoted to a discussion of how the ingredients of cigarette smoke damage the lungs and why we constantly teach, urge, plead, and coerce against the habitual inhalation of cigarette smoke — one of life's most threatening habits.

The 1964 Surgeon General's report on smoking and health clearly indicted smoking as the most important factor in the development of emphysema and bronchitis as well as the other scourge of the lungs, cancer. Thus the prevention of smoking or the cessation of smoking is fundamental for both the prevention and treatment of emphysema and chronic bronchitis. As a matter of record, we feel strongly that much of our program for rehabilitation is hindered, if not entirely neutralized, if one continues to smoke cigarettes.

We will admit straight away that smoking is not the only cause of emphysema and chronic bronchitis. Both diseases were well described in the 1800's before smoking became commonplace; however, during that time both emphysema and chronic bronchitis were very rare. The authors see perhaps one or two patients a year who have either emphysema or chronic bronchitis or both who have never smoked, but the authors see an excess of two hundred new patients a year who have emphysema and chronic bronchitis clearly related to smoking.

Smoking probably damages the lungs by causing inflammation of the alveoli and by causing inflammation of the airways. The inflammatory processes of the alveoli may lead to holes, destruction, and emphysema production, while the inflammatory process of the airways may lead to thickening of the airway lining and obstruction from chronic bronchitis. Whereas we cannot conceive of the repair of the destruction of holes in the alveolar membrane, or the repair of ruptured alveolar walls, it is entirely likely that

27

inflammation of the airways may heal following cessation of smoking. We know, for example, that the irritation of sunburn heals easily. By pulmonary function tests (Chapter I) which measure airflow through the conducting airways, we have measured a reduction in airway obstruction by noting a definite improvement in airflow following the cessation of smoking in some patients.

Smoking may damage the lungs by another mechanism. It has been recently learned through research conducted at a number of medical centers that cigarette smoke can paralyze ciliary activity of the conducting airways. The cilia wave together in a rhythmic fashion to propel mucus out of the depths of the lungs, and into larger air passages where coughing removes the mucus. The cilia beat together like the many oarsmen of rowing canoes to propel the boat down the river. When paralyzed, the cilia do not beat in wave-like form, mucus stagnates and becomes difficult to remove, and the airways become plugged. With the cleansing function paralyzed and almost useless, carcinogens (components of cigarette smoke which are known to cause experimental cancer) are not removed from the lung surface; this may be important in the production of lung cancer.

Emphysema, chronic bronchitis, and lung cancer are related to each other probably through the common denominator of smoking. One of our most courageous patients first came to us with severe chronic bronchitis and a moderately severe degree of emphysema. Respiratory failure (inability of the lungs to provide enough oxygen or remove enough carbon dioxide for life to continue) occurred twice within one month. His life was maintained by a tracheostomy (Chapter X) and breathing was completely supported by a respirator. The patient made a good recovery and with efforts at rehabilitation and continuous oxygen therapy he recovered to the extent that he returned to part-time work. Eight months later, he began suffering from cancer of the lung which has spread widely. He stopped smoking following his second episode of respiratory failure and his chronic bronchitis improved remarkably. It seems so ironic that in spite of stopping the cigarettes which caused his chronic bronchitis, the cigarettes are still able to plague this patient months later because of the lung cancer which was caused by years of cigarette smoking.

We are convinced that smoking is an addiction which has psychological and physical factors. We have seen patients as severely addicted to smoking as one may be addicted to alcohol, barbiturates, or even narcotics. We have had the unfortunate experience of taking care of one poor man who was addicted to heroin. He was an alcoholic and he had smoked cigarettes (four packages each day since the age of seven). An interesting message comes from his life history for it is remarkable that this patient was able to break the dope habit, was ultimately able to stop drinking, but was never able to cease cigarette smoking. In his opinion and on direct questioning, smoking was a much more compelling addiction than either dope or alcohol. This patient developed chronic bronchitis and ultimately died of lung cancer related to smoking.

In referring to smoking, we stress that we are mostly speaking about cigarette smoking. Pipe smokers and cigar smokers who never inhale their smoke do have a slightly increased incidence of bronchitis and emphysema but not nearly as high as cigarette smokers. Pipe and cigar smokers do have an increased incidence of mouth and lip cancer as well. Both pipe and cigar smoking continue to whet the appetite for tobacco and thus, neither are advised generally as a substitute for cigarette smoke. If patients relinquish tobacco completely, gradually the desire to smoke subsides and the urge to douse the lungs with poisons finally ceases.

How To Stop Smoking

Approximately 50 per cent of our patients eventually stop smoking, but we fear that our influence is not what finally helps break the habit. In fact, smoking is such a tremendous addiction for some patients, that we are rarely able to talk these individuals into quitting. We always try, but it takes something more than explanations and more than fear devices (such as showing the patient a lung from a cancer victim or with emphysema or bronchitis who smoked heavily). The addiction to cigarette smoke comes from within. It is an emotional thing and, at times, nothing we say will intellectually convince the patient that he should use all his will power and even superhuman efforts to turn his back on the blackmail of cigarette addiction. Our patients believe what we say, but at first they cannot do anything about it. Often later they can!

Some patients can stop smoking by sheer determination alone. They simply throw their pack away and never smoke another cigarette. At the other end of the spectrum are patients who, we are convinced, can never stop smoking. Fortunately, these latter patients are rare, and total hopeless addiction is not often seen in our clinics. The vast majority of patients have a very considerable difficulty in ceasing smoking. They may try many times to break the habit, but a feeling of nervousness, tobacco hunger, irritability, or emotional upset may return the patient to smoking. Others follow Mark Twain's philosophy, "Stopping smoking is easy; I've done it a thousand times."

In ceasing smoking, the patient must first decide that it is important. He should review his own medical history in terms of symptoms he has learned to tolerate. He should refuse to accept progressive cough, progressive shortness of breath, ultimate disability, and even death from the something that can be avoided. He should confer with his physician, read articles concerning smoking, and view acquaintances, friends, and family around him who are suffering from the disaster of cigarette smoking. It is frequently helpful for the patient to have a goal or set a date on which he will begin to stop or actually stop smoking. This should not be a time of great stress as a time of important business decisions, family decisions, travel, around holidays, etc. Perhaps a weekend when nothing is planned should be set aside for the first period of ceasing smoking. The patient should realize at the outset that in a few hours after "the last cigarette" a feeling of nervousness, a growling stomach, jittery nerves, and irritability may befall him. A substitute may help satisfy some of the craving for smoking. Chewing gum, sucking on life savers, or lemon drops may be helpful. Simply walking outside for fresh air may work. A number of drugs have been advanced to help combat the pangs of cigarette hunger. *Lobeline* is similar to nicotine in its drug action and this drug can be absorbed by mouth. Lobeline is available in over-the-counter preparation by a number of manufacturers (Bantron®, Smoke-eze®, etc.), but studies compared with sugar tablets have not clearly proven the effectiveness of lobeline as an aid in breaking the habit. We have no objection to trying lobeline or any other gimmick which may help the patient succeed in abstaining from tobacco.

One group of patients almost uniformly stops smoking. These are the patients who suffer respiratory failure and whose lives must be completely supported by a respirator. More importantly, these individuals are fighting for their lives and now the strength of their emotion quickly helps curb any appetite for smoke. Afterwards, they are sufficiently frightened by their experience or properly fulfilled with a truly new chance at life that they never want a single cigarette more. It has always seemed a pity to us that man must, at times, suffer the fears of death and even face death before he finally has the strength to save his own life by always providing clean air to the lungs.

After a period of not smoking, most patients learn that the terrible craving for cigarettes comes in waves, but these waves soon subside. Hour by hour, and day by day, the waves become less frequent and less severe. The periods when the patients feel well are lengthened. Soon the craving for tobacco no longer becomes compelling. It may persist for months or even years and may never go away, but it becomes bearable and the feeling for the need of tobacco is replaced by completely new sensations — those of increased pep, energy, and vigor. Cough begins to subside. It may take weeks or months for the cough to go away, but smoking has usually been present for many years and it is natural that some period of time needs to pass for healing of the bronchitis element of the disease to take place. The patient also notices that as his cough ceases, his breathing becomes easier. The patient is able to do more and life takes on a certain new feeling. Once again, the flowers smell and food has a taste and the hairy tongue is gone.

Patients who can stop smoking also develop a certain pride in the knowledge that they have done the most important thing possible to help protect their health. Cancer fears go away and a new feeling of vigor is appreciated.

The authors and our colleagues have recent evidence from research which clearly shows that patients who do stop smoking also stop coughing. We have compared those who stop both smoking and coughing with a similar group of patients who continue to smoke and cough. Our data show that the total life expectancy is measurably increased in those of the first group who stopped both smoking and coughing compared to the continuous smokers. Thus, even though heavy cigarette smoking shortens one's life, some or most of this loss may be prevented by stopping smoking.

What further plea or challenge can we give our readers concerning the smoking problem—we can but offer one of our bits of verse.

Break The Habit
Break the habit,
Or I'll tell the Abbot.
The smoke and fire
Are your funeral pyre.
Eat some stuff
Or chew some snuff.
Mouth some gum
Or suck your thumb.

We sincerely believe that if this book provides no other good than to encourage a few people to stop smoking, our efforts will have been worthwhile.

Air Pollution

The ingredients in the gaseous emissions of industrial chimneys, coal, wood, and oil-burning stoves, incinerators, and the effects of sunlight on automobile exhaust all join forces to produce a haze over our cities and a blaze in our lungs.

Air pollution damages the lungs in a manner much like cigarettes. We find evidence of inflammation as well as spasmodic narrowing of the airways. Air pollution also produces paralysis of the ciliary cleansing mechanism and thus the setup for poor removal of infecting and irritating particles is present. Patients exposed to heavily polluted air suffer more frequent and more severe colds than those not equally exposed.

Sudden disasters such as the famous London and Pennsylvania fogs (smogs) have caused thousands of deaths; here, cause and effect are not doubted. The role of low-grade day-to-day community air pollution on our lungs is much less clear. One scientific study compared the rates and severity of bronchitis in groups of male smokers (Canadian veterans) in four cities. Three cities had significant air pollution and one did not. In spite of heavy smoking in all groups, the group without air pollution fared very much better than those patients from the three cities of severe pollution.

At the present time, we are concerned about air pollution, but we feel smoking is far more important. In a sense both are air pollutions — one is a community problem and the other a personal problem, but both damage the lungs. Cigarette smoking is probably more harmful because the concentrations of smoke are much higher than with atmospheric pollution. Also cigarette smoke bypasses the nose, a most effective filter. Most patients breathe through the nose, nature's filter, when out in the dirty city air.

We are not today advising many patients to move away from the city smog. Perhaps this is advisable, but most of our larger cities have some air pollution and thus unless one moves to the country or a certain few remote cities, air pollution is hard to avoid.

Our affluent society has provided us with the means of destruction of our lungs, and cigarettes are today sold to children, in schools, public buildings, hospitals, and in church basements. With the advent of air pollution, we may call ourselves also the *effluent* society.

Chapter V

Medical Treatment

Numerous drugs are available for the treatment of emphysema and chronic bronchitis. Antibiotics are used to treat infections. A group of drugs called *mucolytic agents* help thin secretions, and anti-inflammatory drugs of the *cortisone* family may be useful in curing the inflammation of some forms of chronic bronchitis. A myriad of bronchodilator drugs are useful in helping to combat spasmodic narrowing of the airways or swelling of the lining of the airways, a phenomenon called bronchospasm, which sometimes occurs with chronic bronchitis or emphysema.

Medical treatment is primarily directed at the element of chronic bronchitis. This is because chronic bronchitis is an inflammatory process of the lining of the airways of the lungs and thus it is possible that inflammation can be reversed and can heal.

Deep chest infections probably begin as a *virus* headcold which ultimately ends in bronchial inflammation and irritation. When this occurs, mucous secretions are markedly increased. At this point in the illness most physicians institute antibiotic therapy. Patients themselves should know when it is time to take this therapy and should report to their physicians when increasing secretions occur, that is, when cough becomes more pronounced or when secretions change from the normal whitish appearance to green, gray or yellow, along with fever. Many physicians give patients a home supply of antibiotics to be taken when these symptoms first begin. This is reasonable because highly effective and safe antibiotics are available which are capable of combating the most common organisms involved in flare-ups of bronchitis. The antibiotic tetracycline is sold under a variety of names including Terramycin®, Achromycin®, and Panmycin®, for examples. This antibiotic is very well tolerated and highly effective against the two most common organisms involved in bronchitis. Considering the fact that attacks of bronchitis probably begin as virus infections, many virus *vaccines* are being studied. At the present time, only influenza virus vaccine is effective and available. Patients with emphysema and chronic bronchitis should receive annual influenza *"boosters"* to help give protection against this one specific form of viral illness which may lead to profound bronchitis or pneumonia. Evidence fails to show that certain bacterial vaccines and "cold shots" are effective.

Many attempts have been made to prevent attacks of bronchitis with the continued *prophylactic* use of antibiotics. Most experts agree that preventative treatment with antibiotics is not effective and thus not worth the expense or bother.

All types of infections and other irritants, can cause inflammation of the airways and an outpouring of secretions (mucus) from the bronchial mucous glands (Chapter III) . These secretions begin to plug the airways and to interfere with the entry and exit of air. Furthermore, these secretions become thick and dried and it is often difficult for patients to cough and clear their airways. For this reason, physicians and nurses direct. their attention toward the humidification and liquefaction of mucus. The best medication for thinning secretions is water. Patients learn to inhale steam by the use of very simple devices or, in some cases, *nebulizers.* In either situation, the aim is toward moist and thin secretions. A very useful device for inhaling steam at home involves the use of a simple baby bottle warmer with steam attachment which directs the steam toward the patient's face (Fig. 14) Steam cools as it reaches the face but provides adequate humidity to thin secretions. Thus, inexpensive equipment (about $5) is available and convenient for home care. Steaming is most effective following bronchodilator therapy. Details of bronchodilator therapy and steaming maneuvers are discussed at length in the chapter on bronchial hygiene (Chapter VI) .

So-called mucolytic drugs also help digest and thus thin *tenacious* mucus. These include the iodides (SSKI) which is taken by drop orally and the more effective inhaled mucolytic agent Mucomyst®.* Since Mucomyst may cause a sore mouth after inhalation, a water or saline mouthwash should be used after each period of inhaling Mucomyst. The mucolytic drugs should be used only for a short period and only when mucus is very thick. Unfortu-

*Mead Johnson.

nately, some patients like to take drugs continuously which have brought relief. Any drug is a two-edged sword and in the case of the mucolytic agents, excessive use may actually cause irritation of the airways.

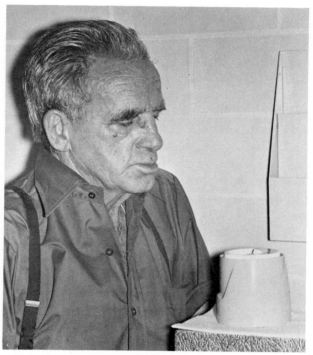

Figure 14. Simple baby bottle warmer with steaming attachment. A column of steam (invisible in Figure) is inhaled by the patient for approximately ten minutes following the inhalation of a bronchodilating drug from a variety of devices including hand bulb nebulizer.

"Bronchospasm" is the sudden constriction of muscular elements of the airways as well as an inflammatory swelling of the lining of the airways. This sudden constriction can cause narrowing of the airways and thus interfere with the exchange of air. Various medications are used to combat this bronchospasm. These include inhaled, Bronchosol®, Adrenalin® and Isuprel®. Drugs can also be taken by mouth or rectally to combat smooth muscle spasm. The most common drugs are aminophylline, given orally or by rectal suppository, and ephedrine, given in a variety of oral preparations (e.g., Amesec®, Quadrinal®, Amodrine®, and Tedral®). Many physicians prefer to use an oral drug three or four times a day, as well as an inhaled bronchodilator, as routine treatment for bronchospasm. This may be effective in a given individual; however, it is likely that bronchospasm is much more common in asthma than in bronchitis and emphysema, and true muscular spasm plays only a small role in the usual case of chronic bronchitis.

It is important for patients to learn to take their bronchodilator drugs in accordance with their individual pattern of disease. For example, if sudden tightening of the chest or wheeze from bronchospasm is felt on exposure to cold air, or on doing normal simple routines such as bathing, then the oral or inhaled bronchodilators may be taken in advance of these events. Also, inhaled bronchodilators may be taken during minor emergencies such as unexplained or excessive shortness of breath while walking or otherwise exercising. Inhaled bronchodilators work more rapidly than oral drugs and are fundamental to a well-conceived home bronchial hygiene program (Chapter VI).

Certain anti-inflammatory drugs, called steroids, are often effective in combating the acute or sudden phase of bronchitis. These drugs must be given by a physician and care must always be exercised since a number of undesirable *side effects,* occasionally serious, may occur with steroid therapy. Steroids are also valuable in a somewhat related disease, bronchial asthma.

In addition to medical therapy directed toward the lungs, physicians may also have to treat heart failure, which may accompany chronic bronchitis or emphysema — a consequence of strain on the heart from low oxygenation or carbon dioxide build-up. Digitalis and *diuretics* are helpful to induce the kidneys to excrete the salt and water which often accumulate during the development of heart failure.

It should be stressed that literally hundreds of drugs are available to treat emphysema and chronic bronchitis. These drugs may bear many similarities and the mechanisms of action are basically four: the relief of muscle spasm; the reversal of inflammation; the combating of *edema,* and the thinning of secretions. Thus far, no drug is a *panacea,* nothing can be considered curative and we must regard our drugs as simple but useful tools in the management of emphysema and chronic bronchitis today.

We personally do not use a large variety of drugs for the above reason. All too often we encounter the situation which plagued a middle-aged machinist patient of ours. At bedtime, he would take a *sedative* to sleep (sedatives are dangerous in patients with serious emphysema or chronic bronchitis), on arising in the morning he would take a "pep pill" to wake him up because of *somnalence* or too little oxygen from too little breathing because of the sedative. The day followed with appetite stimulants (generally ineffective), oral bronchodilators, taken three to four times a day, cortisone (which continually upset his stomach), medicines to quiet the stomach, inhaled bronchodilators, antidepressant drugs followed by tranquilizers, antibiotics at the first sign or thought of a cold, digitalis and diuretics for swollen ankles, aminophylline by rectum, laxatives for constipation, and followed next day by remedies for loose bowels and on and on. This particular patient was markedly improved within two days after cessation of nearly all of these mutually opposing drugs. Following re-education, simple methods of bronchial hygiene and exercise training, a much happier, healthier, and financially secure patient emerged.

Chapter VI

Bronchial Hygiene

IN EARLIER CHAPTERS we have described inflammation of the airways (Chapter I and III), that is enlargement and thickening of the mucous glands contained in the walls of the airways and excessive mucus produced by these irritated airways. This chapter is designed to explain the need for and the means of clearing the airways of secretions and combating irritation. We prefer the term bronchial hygiene because it is descriptive and explains what we want to do. To paraphrase our intent, we might have well entitled this chapter "How to be Nice to the Lungs." The cessation of all smoking must be the first step!

In more specific terms, bronchial hygiene includes all measures we use to clear the airways of irritation and secretions. Bronchial hygiene includes everything that is done in inhalation therapy in our institution. This is the backbone of medical treatment, exercise, and the rehabilitation program.

From a scientific standpoint, we are trying to get maximum dilation of the airways and decongestion of the airway lining (Chapter V). In a sense, the bronchodilators (Bronchosol,® Isuprel and Vaponefrin®) work in similar fashion to nose drops or nasal *decongestants*. Nose drops shrink and reduce the swelling of the nasal passageway. After this, the next step is to provide moisture to the airways so that the dry thick mucus may be moisturized and the reluctant secretions then become vulnerable to expulsion by coughing.

Nebulization Therapy

The first step in a proper bronchial hygiene program is effective nebulization of bronchodilators deep into the conducting airways. The most common bronchodilators in general use are Bronchosol,® Isuprel, Vaponefrin, and Aerolone®. These are closely related drugs which act on the lining of the airways, the bronchial mucosa, to shrink and thus combat congestion of these conducting airways. Some of the deposited medication is also absorbed and the medication may affect other organs. One will feel palpitations or a rapid heart beat if excessive medicine is absorbed. The absorbed drug, however, may combat muscular spasm to a degree, so some absorption is probably beneficial.

The medications should rarely, if ever, be used undiluted. We routinely tell our patients to dilute ten drops of bronchodilator with twenty drops of water, giving a 1:2 dilution. This usually provides more than enough mixture for each period of nebulization. When considerable mixture remains at the end of the nebulization period, we advise five drops of medication and ten drops of water, which is the same concentration. The unused material should be discarded after each treatment period.

Many different types of nebulizers are available. All of these have the ability to produce tiny airborne particles of drug or moisture which is inhaled deep into the lungs. The small *particle size* is essential to proper distribution of medication. Larger particles land ("rain out") in the larger airways (trachea and bronchi) . Smaller particles deposit on the smaller airway branches while the very tiniest particles do not settle at all and are simply exhaled. All nebulizers need a source of power to compress air across the jet assembly. The impact of compressed air forces medication against the jet and this is what breaks the liquid into the various sizes of droplets. The very largest drops actually "rain out" within the nebulizer and only the *respirable sized particles* which are small enough to be carried into the lungs effect bronchodilation.

A variety of methods can be used to deliver compressed air into the nebulizer assembly. By far, the most common method is the simple rubber or plastic bulb. With each squeeze a puff of air provides good nebulization. The two most popular hand bulb nebulizers are illustrated in Figure 15 [DeVilbiss #42 (left) and #40 (right)].

The hand bulb nebulizer is entirely satisfactory for many patients. Their use does require some muscular strength and coordination and, above all, the patient must be completely instructed in the proper use of the nebulizer. In brief, the patient is instructed to empty his lungs as much as possible and then to inhale slowly as the hand bulb is squeezed with a fairly forceful effort.

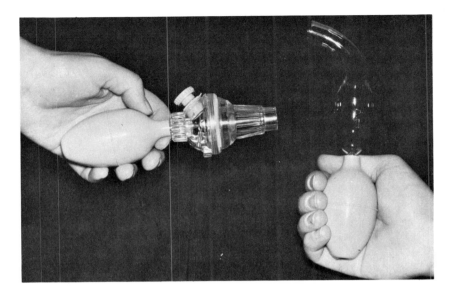

Figure 15. Two commonly used hand bulb nebulizers, DeVilbiss #42 on the left and DeVilbiss
#40 on the right. Both of these nebulizers can be
used by other powered devices.

The nebulizer is positioned at the mouth with the mouth slightly
open. The lips or teeth should not grasp the end of the nebulizer.
The reason for this is that the patient must be able to draw in
additional air to be able to deliver the medication deep to the
lungs. After inhaling, the patient should pause momentarily in
order to allow the medication to deposit. Exhalation against
slightly pursed lips in the manner used in breathing training
(Chapter VIII) may also allow for better distribution and deposi-
tion of the inhaled drug.

Some patients have difficulty coordinating the "squeeze and
breathe" sequence of the hand bulb nebulizer. For these individuals, simple and inexpensive pumps or excellent air com-
pressors can be used.

One of the most popular pump-driven nebulizers is shown in
Figure 16. This device sells for approximately fifty dollars and pro-

vides the work of neubulization. It adds a measure of convenience to today's care. When one considers the lifelong nature of disease and daily requirements for bronchial hygiene, devices similar to this seem valuable and realistic from the standpoint of cost. Simple foot pumps and bicycle pumps can also be used, but they are somewhat less convenient and are not commonly available commercially.

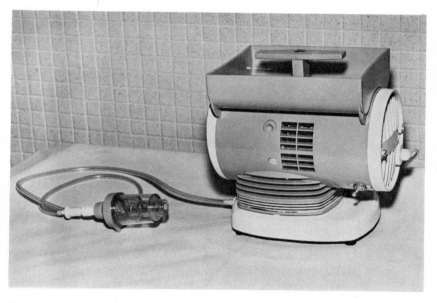

Figure 16. Simple pump-driven nebulizer which is extremely convenient to use. Cost is approximately fifty dollars.

If the patient has oxygen in the home, the nebulizer can be attached to the oxygen tank at the flowmeter for a source of pressure. This also works well for hospitalized patients since the oxygen line in most hospital rooms fits a flowmeter which with tubing and a "Y" tube assembly provides fine nebulization.

Instruction of bronchial hygiene requires sufficient time for the patient to understand exactly what is intended. These instructions are often efficiently provided by nurse specialists or inhalation therapists in small group sessions (Fig. 17). Also, individual instruction is useful in emphasizing points in care as well as the specific prescription ordered by each patient's own physician (Fig. 18).

Cleaning the Nebulizer

The nebulizer should be cleaned frequently to prevent contamination and multiplication of bacteria which occasionally may occur within the nebulizer. Our method of home cleaning and sterilization is as follows:

Instructions:

The daily care of the nebulizer is part of the bronchial hygiene program. The main reason for bronchial hygiene is to clean out the lungs; thus it is important to use a clean nebulizer for this ritual. Washing in soap and water and rinsing with hot water will suffice for the daily or twice daily cleansing. It is a good idea to soak the entire glass part in a 1:6

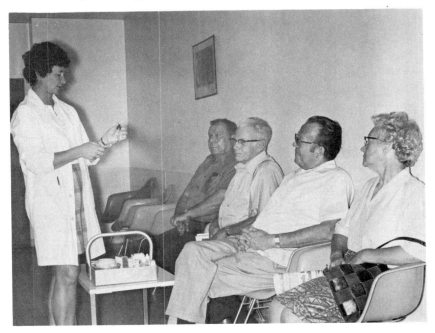

Figure 17. Group instruction by nurse–inhalation-therapist. Patients are taught details of bronchial hygiene and self-care.

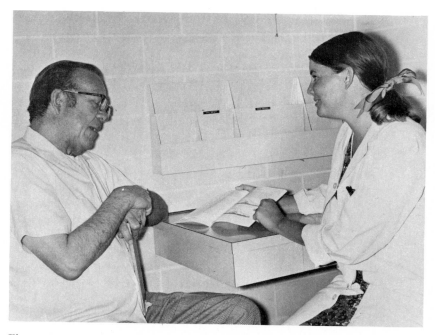

Figure 18. Individual instruction by physiotherapist using this patient care manual.

solution of vinegar and water twice a week. This will destroy an organism commonly found in inhalation equipment.

In patients who simply cannot take a deep breath due to exceedingly severe obstruction of the airways, something more than a hand bulb or powered nebulizer is needed. In these cases, IPPB machines are useful.

A simple hand-held IPPB device is entirely adequate for most cases. This device, the Hand-E-Vent (Fig. 19), has the same capabilities of more complicated automatic devices. The pressure source powers not only the nebulizer but also the device within the handle (Venturi) which increases flow. The device has been extremely useful in the past four years in providing home IPPB therapy and can be mastered by the patient himself. He therefore becomes independent of technicians, nurses or physicians' assistance and certainly does not require a trip to the doctors office or clinic for

IPPB treatments. This device and others is available for approximately $150.

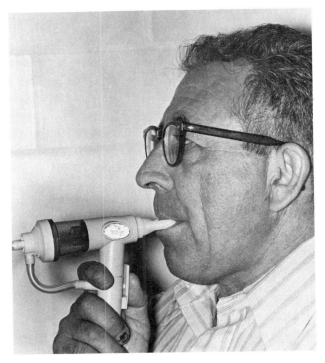

Figure 19. Simple hand-held pressure breathing device (Hand-E-Vent, Ohio Medical Products, Madison, Wisconsin). Patient compresses flap valve in right hand and allows pressure generated by power source to fill the lungs to a comfortable level of inhalation and then release of right hand (thumb) allows exhalation through machine. Several deep breaths (approximately 6-10 per minute) promote the delivery of a bronchodilating drug.

The most popular form of nebulization today is the metered dose device which gives a measured "puff" of nebulized bronchodilator (Fig. 20). The medication is carried in a small can attached to a small plastic device which directs the spray into the open mouth, similar to the manner in which the hand bulb or pump driven nebulizer is used. These are pocket-sized devices.

They have tremendous value from the standpoint of ease of use and portability. Their only drawback is that most of the medication is delivered in large particles. Current evidence suggests that with these large droplets, little medication gets down to the smaller airways where medication is also needed. Another drawback is the high concentration of medication in the metered dose device. This concentration may be excessive so that it is possible for irritation to result when used too often. For this reason, we still prefer the conventional nebulizers described earlier in this chapter. We also prescribe the metered dose devices for the patient to carry with him to work and play.

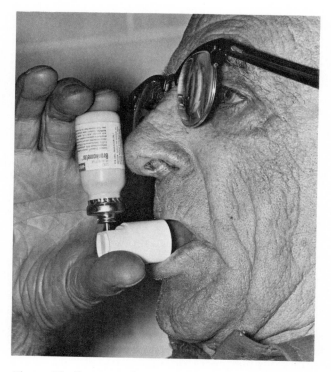

Figure 20. Compressed metered dose device convenient for inhalation of bronchodilating aerosol (Bronkosol®).

We must warn here against the excessive use of any nebulized bronchodilator. Excessive use may render the drug ineffective.

The drugs may be used to the extent that the airways simply will not respond any longer. If this occurs, we have lost an important drug for bronchospasm.

Worse than this, however, excessive use of nebulized bronchodilator may lead to the so-called "rebound phenomenon." After the drug wears off, the mucous membrane may be more congested than ever before. This also occurs in the excessive use of nose drops. One gets into a vicious cycle of excessive medication followed by rebound congestion and then the patient will once again take excessive medication to overcome the rebound and on and on!

Moisture

After nebulization of *aerosolized* medication, the next step in bronchial hygiene is the delivery of moisture into the lungs to wet and thin secretions. Numerous humidifiers are available. These are both simple and cheap as well as elaborate and expensive. The purpose of all these devices is to moisten the air that the patient inhales. Some equipment utilizes the nebulization principle and water is broken into inhalable particles which can be delivered into the lungs. Others simply saturate the air with humidity. Heated humidifiers may be more effective because warm air can carry more moisture than cold air.

There is tremendous variation among patients with chronic respiratory disease concerning the tolerance and acceptability of warm moisture. Many asthmatics and a few patients with chronic bronchitis will feel "choked up" while breathing warm moisture but will be able to inhale cool mist effectively. The reverse may also be the case and warm mist may be preferred. Physicians allow patients to inhale moisture by whatever means is best tolerated. The important thing is to get adequate moisture into the lungs.

Good general hydration is also important and thus, patients should be instructed to drink large quantities of water each day. Probably two to three quarts of water should be consumed while awake in order to insure good general hydration of all the tissues, particularly the lungs. One of our physician colleagues teaches her patients to check on inadequate hydration by simply having them observe the color of the urine stream. If it is too yellow, it is too concentrated (not enough water) and the patient then knows to start drinking water until his urine becomes colorless.

Clearing the Lungs

The whole purpose of the bronchial hygiene program is to clear the lungs of secretions. Thus it does little good to nebulize and inhale steam unless the secretions thus mobilized can be expectorated. The simple act of controlled and coordinated coughing will in most cases remove secretions. Some parts of the lungs are more effectively drained by gravity with the patient in certain positions and these positions are listed briefly in Figures 21, 22, 23, and 24. It often helps to pound upon the back with *cupped hands* (Fig. 25) to help vibrate and loosen sections for removal by coughing.

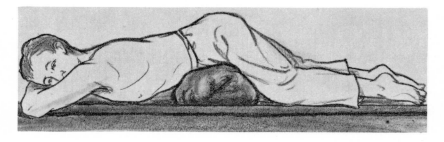

Figure 21. Patient now in position for postural drainage. Drains portion of lower lobe.

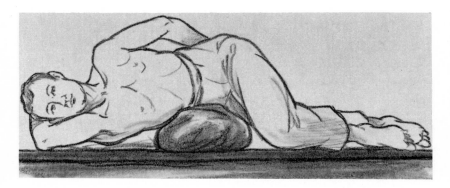

Figure 22. Lying on right side to drain left lower lung.

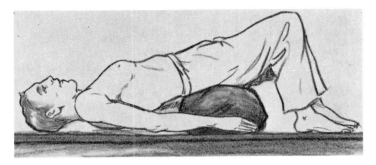

Figure 23. Lying on back to drain anterior (front) portion of chest.

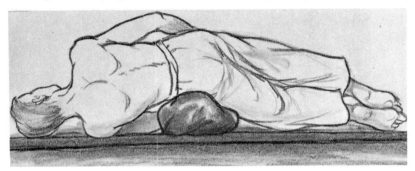

Figure 24. Lying on left side to drain right lung.

The use of gravity to help drain the lungs is called *postural drainage*. When we are erect, our upper lobes drain by gravity. The middle lobe and lingula (equivalent of the middle lobe on the left) and the lower lobes are best drained by certain special positions in bed. For example, some areas of the lungs are best drained in the face-down position with the head somewhat lower than the feet. Lying on one's side or on the back with the head lower than the feet also helps drain other portions of the lung segments. If postural drainage is used to clear the airways, this should always be performed after both nebulizing with a bronchodilator (Such as Bronchosol®) and steaming. One should lie in each position for ten minutes or so, or until secretions are produced. By practice, one will learn how long it takes in each position to clear accumulated secretions. A minute or two in one position may suffice while ten to fifteen minutes may be needed for another posture in order to drain a particularly difficult segment of the lung. Drainage is best performed on an empty stomach. Occasionally the cough which is stimulated by the nebulized secretions will cause stomach upset, nausea and vomiting.

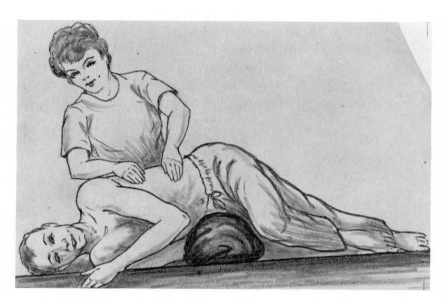

Figure 25. Pounding on chest with cupped hands to vibrate and loosen secretions in the various postural drainage positions (Figs. 21, 22, 23, and 24).

Postural drainage may be performed while using oxygen. In patients who need IPPB for nebulization, drainage may be aided by simultaneous use of the pressure breather. The forced inspiration allows the patient to take a breath and thus force air deep into the lungs and behind plugs of mucus. The cough or forced expiration which may follow the deep inspiration will help force out stubborn secretions. Some physicians have advised against the use of IPPB when the secretion problem is severe for fear of forcing the mucus further out into the lungs by the force of the pressure breather. This does not happen because the airways enlarge on inspiration and reduce in diameter on expiration. Thus, the forced inspiration in a sense opens the airways and allows air to flow past the thickened secretions. When the airways become smaller on expiration, the plugs of secretions may tend to occlude the airways but force of the returning air propels the secretions outward into the large airways where a coordinated expulsive cough will allow expectoration.

Bronchial hygiene should be performed at least each morning and evening. The morning treatment will help remove the secretions which were accumulated while sleeping. The evening period will provide maximum clearing so that the patient hopefully will not be awakened with as much coughing at night. Bronchial hygiene may be needed at other times during the day. Each patient has his own pattern which can be followed in coordination with normal daily living. During chest colds, nebulization of medications and water may have to be done many times because of markedly increased mucus production.

At first, some patients have difficulty adjusting to what they regard as a complicated ritual. While the practice of bronchial hygiene should be compulsively and meticulously followed, we know from experience that this can be done efficiently and within a reasonable period of time. The time spent is a very good investment. One may wish to nebulize only three to four minutes with a bronchodilator. Approximately ten minutes of steaming usually will provide considerable moisture and controlled coughing or a short period of postural drainage — maybe only five to six minutes — may suffice to clear the airways. This whole process should take no more than twenty to twenty-five minutes each time.

It should be stressed that each patient will learn to "feel the need" for bronchial hygiene and also each patient will eventually learn when he has achieved maximum cleaning of the airways. In performing bronchial hygiene, it is much more important to "go by the feel" rather than measure each treatment by the clock. A few patients become too compulsive and literally spend hours cleansing their lungs. One patient of ours, a very successful and busy businessman would take ten minutes to prepare his medication just so, nebulize bronchodilator fifteen to twenty minutes, followed by twenty to thirty minutes steaming and another thirty to forty-five minutes in the various positions of postural drainage.

At the time, the whole "ceremony" as he called it took two hours to perform. He had to get up early to do it before leaving for work. He was getting to work later and becoming discouraged. After going over his program with more instructions, we convinced him that bronchial hygiene should take no more than twenty to twenty-five minutes each time. He gradually became more efficient and finally learned to adjust his program to a normal daily routine.

We conclude this chapter by stressing that the bronchial hygiene program, tremendously important and the true cornerstone of medical management, is rendered ineffective if the patients continue to smoke cigarettes. What we are trying to do is clear the lungs of secretions that plug the airways. Smoking as well as air pollution continue to produce irritation and thus secretions. Needless to say, when infections are causing secretions, the infection should also be treated (Chapter V).

Chapter VII

Breathing Machines

In recent years, an increasing number of machines capable of supporting breathing by providing work to inflate the lungs have become available. It is of great interest to review the history of the development of the various breathing machines in common use today. The basic valve for the first generally-used breathing machine was developed in the mid-forties by physicians and engineers involved in high-altitude aviation problems, because at that time the airplanes were not pressurized. With astronauts reaching the moon, some of these problems faced by aviation researchers in the mid-forties seem trivial, but one should recall that in the mid-forties, a fighter pilot could not ascend to above 37,000 feet because even 100 per cent oxygen breathing would not provide normal oxygenation. It was necessary at altitudes above 37,000 feet to force oxygen under pressure into the patient's lungs in order to achieve normal oxygenation of the blood. To provide for pressure breathing, some means of a demand valve which could work in inspiration and expiration was needed. Two basic valves emerged (Bennett and Burns valves) which would allow for the inflow of air during inspiration and no inward flow of air during expiration. These proved to be entirely acceptable in the pressure breathing of high-altitude aircraft and, following the war, found application as the central valve mechanism for a variety of breathing machines. At the present time, only twenty-five years later, some fifty companies produce several-hundred different machines of various sizes, shapes, capabilities, and cost. The intent of this chapter is to discuss, in simple terms, the role of breathing machines in the care of emphysema and bronchitis patients and to give guidelines concerning the utility of these machines and their safe operation in the home.

All of the machines in common use today are called intermittent positive-pressue breathing devices, abbreviated IPPB. Most of these machines cause a flow of air into the lungs until the

machine's preset pressure is reached in the lungs and airways. At
this point, the machine shuts off and exhalation occurs passively
and usually against no back pressure. Most of these devices can be
so adjusted that a very mild respiratory effort will initiate inspiration and airflow into the lungs will occur until the pressure in the
lungs equals the machine's pressure, whereupon a valve closes and
the flow of air stops. Exhalation then occurs passively until another effort opens the valve and forced fresh air again floods the
lungs. Somewhat similar devices do not have the automatic-valve-
type mechanism and the patient simply uses his thumb to cover
a port which then allows air to flow into the lungs; the thumb
can be released when the patient feels his lungs are fully inflated
(see Chapter 6). These devices have the advantages of being simpler
and less expensive. They require more patient participation in
their use, but this is no disadvantage since patients who have such
devices in their homes should be fully trained and adept in the use
of their home equipment. A commonly-used commercial home machine is illustrated in Figure 26. The primary purpose is to force
nebulized medication and water into the lungs. Whereas breathing
machines are exceedingly effective in the delivery of drugs and
water, these agents can be delivered by simpler devices in many
cases (Chapter VI). Only those patients who cannot take a large
enough breath to deliver medication because of limited lung function need complicated machines to deliver medications.

We should entitle this paragraph "Everybody Doesn't Need
One." This refers to the nearly mass demand for home IPPB
machines for patients who have chronic bronchitis and emphysema. Actually, and to repeat, the sole purpose of an IPPB
machine is to do the work of delivering medication and to provide
some temporary relief from the work of breathing during short
periods while one is allowing the machine to toil. It is also possible
that machines improve the distribution of drug delivery in severely
obstructed patients.

Our recent experience shows that anyone who can naturally
draw medications into his own lungs from a powered nebulizer or
humidifier does not need something to do this work for him. We do
not prescribe home IPPB machines for everyone. We select the individual who moves very little air and who needs good nebuliza-

tion of both medications and steam in the home. For this individual we do prescribe a home device and recognize that the primary
disadvantage of the currently available automatic home devices is
their considerable expense. Less-expensive devices are now available (Chapter VI).

We should comment on the office or clinic use of IPPB
machines. Except for instruction in the physician's office or a
clinic, therapy with the IPPB machine should not be a doctor's
office or clinic procedure but should be performed in the home,
if the patient is in need of IPPB as an outpatient. This fact seems
eminently obvious to us because of the simple fact that if a
patient needs a powered nebulizer, he needs it all the time. Thus,
he needs it either in the hospital or the home. Trips to the
doctor's office or clinic are time-consuming and expensive. How
much better it would be to teach the patient to use his own IPPB
machine in the home under a physician's supervision.

Chapter VI was devoted in part to advice on how to use
simple devices for the delivery of medications. The remainder of
this chapter will explain the use of conventional IPPB machines
in the home.

IPPB machines are often used at a driving pressure of 12 to 15
centimeters of water, and the pressure delivered into the lungs is
registered on the gauge found on most of the IPPB units. Some
patients can learn to take 18, 20, even 25 centimeters pressure,
in order to take even larger breaths and thus deliver important
medication and water to distant and diseased areas of the lung.
In using the machine, the patient should allow the device to fill
the lungs with no resistance. When the preset pressure is reached,
the valve will shut off automatically. In machines that require the
patient to release the pressure delivery by thumb, the inflow of air
will have to be stopped by thumb release when the preset pressure
is reached on a dial or when the patient's lungs have a feeling of
fullness.

One of the most common devices in use today in the home
is the Bennett home model (Fig. 26). The principle for all
of these machines is the same. To repeat, the patient's inspiratory
effort triggers a valve to open and air enters the lungs under
pressure delivering the prescribed medication and moisture. Pressure developing in the lungs finally shuts off the valve and a port

opens to allow passive (relaxed) expiration. Treatment periods usually last ten-to-fifteen minutes, three or four times a day. Patients can be taught to use these machines more often in certain situations such as a sudden shortness of breath, for periods of drowsiness, and for more effective nebulization during flare-ups of infection.

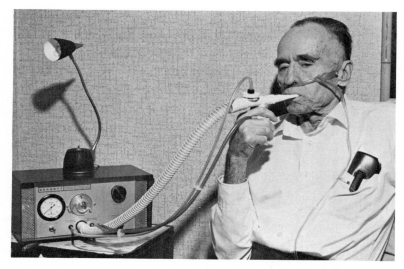

Figure 26. Patient using automatic pressure breathing machine at home (Bennett AP-5). This device has the advantage of being automatic. Note patient also receiving oxygen by double nasal prongs similar to Figure 29.

In these situations the machine is "something to turn to." Very often, difficult plugs of mucus will be mobilized. Coughing may fail to remove these plugs and the patient needs an assisting device. By relieving the patient of the work of breathing, he can often recover from severe breathlessness and remain comfortable using the machine for a time.

Care of Home Machines

Proper care and sterilization of home machines is important. The nebulizer devices and each piece of equipment can become contaminated with bacteria. These multiply and can be forced into the lung, possibly causing trouble.

At least once a week, the tubing and nebulizer assembly should be removed and washed with soap and water. Next, the tubing and nebulizer should be soaked in a bleach solution such as Clorox for ten minutes and then rinsed with water. Attention to this simple procedure will keep the home machine clean, safe, and attractive, since staining from medications will be removed by the bleach. The machine should be used only by the patient and not tried by visitors, others with respiratory ailments, or family members.

Much emotional and considerable financial investment has been attached to these breathing machines. Many opponents and proponents have gathered forces or have contradicted each other in the sport of "who has the best machine?" We do not support one or another device but recognize that "ventilation is ventilation" by whatever method. Many patients with machines may not need them at all and the machine certainly should not and must not replace the rest of medical care although, unfortunately, this is often the case.

The poetic amongst us have composed the following as a matter of fact and record.

My Apparatus

My apparatus
Can't change my status
But when I'm blue
It helps my pO_2.
Its rhythmic pumps
Are like grinds and bumps
But it's all I have left to do.

So sad — we prefer the following:

Ode To An IPPB

I think I wish I'd never see
Another damn IPPB
A box adorned with knobs and dials
But one which can't replace the smiles
Of my love and I alone
When I could breathe upon my own.

The above liberally endowed with both pathos and love are important to consider, for the machines should help medical care, be a vehicle of medication, be something to use in distress, but should not tie patients inside the home and away from visits, friends, and normal happy living. When visiting and lecturing in another city not long ago, we talked to a patient who had a home breathing device. This patient was kind enough to participate in a program we were giving on emphysema and bronchitis. In spite of his good humor and relative vigor, he believed he had to cut short the visit and hurry home to his breathing machine. He really did not need it, but he stopped everything and ran home to his gadget.

The most significant purpose of breathing machines is to support patients' lives during respiratory failure. Conventional devices already described and somewhat more complicated equipment can be used in acute hospital situations to support breathing. These machines support life while doctors and nurses work together to treat and remedy what is known as respiratory failure. Respiratory failure occurs when the lungs, in disease, are unable to provide enough oxygenation and remove enough CO_2 for life to exist. Respiratory failure may occur in emphysema, chronic bronchitis, or a variety of other illnesses. In the care and management of respiratory failure the machines are essential.

In respiratory failure, the machines are usually connected to a tracheostomy, a tube which is placed directly into the trachea (see Chapter X), or to an endotracheal tube which is placed either through the mouth or through the nose into the trachea.

These machines can support life for many days while therapeutic efforts are directed toward treating the underlying reversible factors in the disease, which include the infection, secretion problem, bronchospasm, and any associated heart failure. In a sense, these machines gain time in order that other therapeutic maneuvers may work. Certainly, the development of breathing machines has been a tremendous advance in the acute care of patients with emphysema and bronchitis. These machines have provided for long-term survival for many patients. We were reminded of this recently when we saw one of our earlier patients whose life was supported for five days with a breathing machine to allow for aggressive medical treatment. We were called to see this individual when the physician in charge believed that death was imminent.

Following a tracheostomy and removal of tremendous obstructing secretions, the patient regained consciousness while the machine supported his life. After five days of tracheostomy and support of breathing, the patient could breathe without the machine and the tracheostomy was closed. Over the next two months he made a remarkable recovery, gained weight, and returned to work. He is still living, five years later, and has never had another hospitalization. Of course, his improvement was based upon more than machinery. He received intensive medical and nursing care, stopped smoking, and began to take a new interest in life and a new interest in normal activity. He was proud of himself when he returned to work. But the point to be made here is that we absolutely needed the machine for a few days in order to gain precious time for our therapeutic efforts to succeed.

The newest of the respirators for intensive care is shown in Figure 27. In the first edition of this book this machine was discussed in the last chapter on the "Outlook and the Future." Now this device is generally available throughout the country and abroad and has saved many lives!

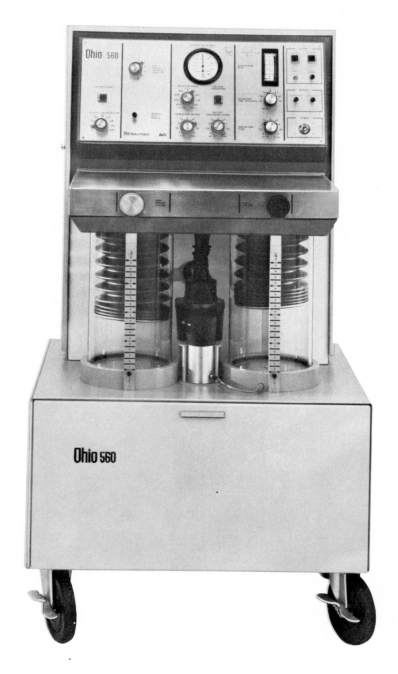

Figure 27. New ventilator for intensive care and recovery room. (Ohio 560, Ohio Medical Products Co., Madison, Wisconsin)

Chapter VIII

Physical Reconditioning

THIS CHAPTER IS DEVOTED TO the use of physical measures to improve breathing performance and efficiency. These goals are achieved by means of breathing retraining and graded general exercises which are designed to increase endurance and exercise efficiency. Since much of the disability of both emphysema and chronic bronchitis involves a damaged mechanism of breathing and since much effort and work of breathing is wasted in discoordinated breathing efforts, breathing retraining can provide increased comfort. Reliance on an efficient breathing pattern may be a real comfort when attacks of sudden increased shortness of breath occur for no known reason or during essential, but somewhat excessive exercise.

Patients with severe obstruction to airflow in either emphysema or chronic bronchitis are frequently laboring to breathe, but may be accomplishing very little. The prime muscles used in the act of normal respiration are the strong respiratory muscles (intercostals, i.e. the muscles between the ribs — Chapter I), the pectoral or upper chest muscles, and the all-important diaphragm. Other muscles come into play during labored breathing; these are the neck and abdominal muscles. Use of the neck muscles during inspiration really does little good and only makes the patient tense. The neck muscles can only elevate the chest a little and the fully inflated chest is already maximally elevated. Thus this sort of effort is wasted.

In desperation, some patients give a sort of grunt by contracting their abdominal muscles as they labor to get a little more air in. Contraction of the abdominal muscles is really an expiratory effort and the grunt and passage of intestinal gas prove it. The abdominal muscles are useful in respiration but they should be relaxed on inspiration and only on expiration are they of use in forcing air out of the the lungs in a coordinated expiratory effort.

To review, the basic *physiologic* (functional) problem in both

61

emphysema and chronic bronchitis is getting used air out of the lungs so new fresh air can be taken in. In emphysema and chronic bronchitis, both of the lungs are overinflated and a dilemma occurs when the fully distended lungs are unable to take in new fresh air. The whole idea of breathing retraining is to learn how to empty the lungs more efficiently and effectively in a coordinated relaxed manner so that new air can be inhaled. For this reason, the emphasis is placed on expiration. Expiration should take place over as long a period of time as possible. Patients should learn to relax their abdominal muscles and let their belly become *protuberant* during inspiration so that the diaphragm, the main breathing muscle, can descend to a maximum degree. During expiration, the abdominal muscles should contract very gently in order to help expel air from the inflated lungs. All too often, patients are contracting their belly muscles during inspiration, but this is an expiratory effort and may in fact interfere with the movement of air as we said earlier. The neck muscles are of no use in breathing and should always be relaxed during coordinated breathing. Patients need to learn to exhale slowly against slightly pursed lips very much as one begins to whistle. It is possible that breathing against a mild resistance helps keep airways from collapsing (Chapter II) and this helps remove additional air. Exhalation should be performed at first with the patient's hands on the lower chest and abdomen so that the patient feels the abdominal muscles contracting during exhalation. In this way, one can begin to learn coordinated breathing in expiration and inspiration can then follow rather automatically and effortlessly. Sometimes a counting sequence helps, three even counts for inhalation and 5, 6, 7 even counts for expiration, so that expiration is at least twice as long as inspiration. It is stressed that if the lungs can be emptied in a relaxed fashion, perhaps an increased amount of fresh air can enter the lungs. This breathing pattern is learned by the patients themselves or taught by physical therapists, nurses, and physicians.

Some patients have trouble learning this rather reversed breathing pattern at first. As a matter of fact, we are really asking and training our patients to "breathe in reverse." They are urged to forget the labor of inspiration and thus relax their abdomen. They need to concentrate on expiration and let the intake of new air occur rather automatically. Patients do well at first, but then forget and thus they need repeated instruction by their physician, nurse, or physical therapist (Fig. 28). Practice and more practice will eventually gain the art. For example: One patient was given extensive breathing training and spent many hours learning the whys and hows of emphysema and bronchitis care — he seemed a most intelligent man, most ready to learn. During the training sessions he did the pattern beautifully, yet on visits to the patient's room, he would become anxious and dyspneic. Close observation of the patient indicated a complete lack of coordination during a normal life experience (talking). The relaxed reassuring therapist reviewed the fundamental principle of breathing retraining which the patient had forgotten. A reminder was all this

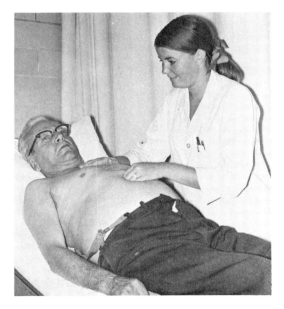

Figure 28. Physiotherapist stressing relaxation of abdomen (left hand) and accessory muscles (right hand) during inspiration. Expiration is then forceful, promoting emptying of the lungs.

man needed. During the rest of the visit, the gentleman breathed the "new way" and talked at length without becoming dyspneic.

Once it is well established, this coordinated breathing program can be continued while exercising and even continued during sleep. Many people feel relief of their symptoms during breathing retraining. To summarize, breathing retraining probably works by improving coordination and thus efficiency and perhaps by strengthening the muscles of respiration. The new pattern does not strengthen the lungs themselves, but many people feel marked relief of symptoms with the new breathing pattern.

General Physical and Muscular Reconditioning

A general physical retraining and reconditioning program is fundamental to rehabilitation in emphysema and chronic bronchitis. Patients who are chronically ill with a disease which interferes with breathing frequently become more and more sedentary. These patients lose interest in previously enjoyed activities, sit at home and do nothing, and all their muscles become wasted and flabby. In truth, the patient is "out of shape." It is known through recent research that even chronically ill patients can be improved by a graded exercise program. It is likely that these exercises improve breathing efficiency and this can be compared to spring training periods which athletes utilize to get "in shape." Studies from our laboratories and those of other researchers show that patients can exercise and walk farther at a slower pulse rate, a slower respiratory rate, and with the need for lesser amounts of oxygen than before being retrained. Patients may gain weight during physical reconditioning.

After the new breathing pattern is learned, the patient should continue to walk using the same controlled breathing pattern. One should walk at a slow pace in a relaxed fashion and should walk to the limits of tolerance. It should be stressed that a mild and moderate shortness of breath is not harmful and does not mean that the lungs are being damaged. Even very healthy people who engage in strenuous exercise feel shortness of breath which is appropriate for exercise, and these symptoms, of course, go away when exercise is discontinued. This is also true of patients with emphysema and chronic bronchitis. Shortness of breath which subsides on stopping or sitting is in no way harmful. Patients need a gradually increasing program so that they walk greater distances an increasing number of times each day. This can be done by having a goal within the room, within the house, in the yard, or up the block. Go to the same place each time and then a little farther. Stop when shortness of breath occurs and then continue. Take the same exercise or stroll more frequently each day. Begin with stairsteps after you walk a block. Above all, continue the exercise program in force without interruption and with the idea that you will never be entirely satisfied with your ability to walk a given distance. We have learned that even very ill patients can do a little more each day and actually no real limit is usually reached, even though patients are measured to walk farther each day for several months or years. When one can walk far enough for normal daily living, at least one of the objectives of the exercise program has been reached. Some patients prefer to buy a *pedometer* which measures their "mileage" during each day of exercise.

More seriously ill patients may be so short of breath that even sitting in a chair leaves them breathless. These patients may need oxygen both to relieve the breathlessness of a sedentary existence and also to provide oxygen for the oxygen cost of exercising. Patients can begin to walk around the room with oxygen, from the conventional metal cylinder and increase their exercise by these means. Some oxygen tanks can be equipped with wheels (Chapter VII) and thus portable oxygen supply is possible. As listed in Chapter IX, liquid oxygen "walkers" are available within a limited number of centers. These are ideal to provide oxygen for the exercise breathing program. These new oxygen devices are becoming generally available now. They are effective in providing for increased activity in patients with severe emphysema and chronic bronchitis (see Chapter IV).

Physicians may exercise patients on a treadmill or stationary bicycle in the hospital. This is for convenience and to show the degree of improvement in the cold statistics of feet walked or minutes walked. We have seen one rugged individual improve from twenty to twenty-five feet per day to literally five to six miles a day on the treadmill. Although the patient was impressed, and so were our statistical experts, his new ability really meant something when he could return home. Then he could replace the squeals and roar of the treadmill with the afternoon breeze and the flowers of his yard. He walked to friends' homes two blocks away rather than the three hundred treadmill yards. Rehabilitation is not designed to please the record book of the physician scientist; it is designed to get the patient home to normal living.

We have used the term "spring training" because it likens the situation of our flabby chronic emphysema and bronchitis patients with the out-of-shape athlete ready for spring training. We adopted this term several springs ago when a fifty-five-year-old housewife, who had been in and out of several hospitals for four months and in bed all of the time, came in to our hospital in transfer. Her case was that of bronchitis and heart strain (cor pulmonale) and was marked by complications. Lack of will prevailed because of the chronic illness. Exercise made possible by continuous oxygen finally succeeded in giving her confidence and strength and gradually she progressed to the chair, to ambulating around the room, and finally she went home with oxygen. She has increased her activity gradually over the next eighteen months; she was fully active within her own home and could walk a block outside whenever she wanted.

To conclude, breathing retraining may do much to reduce the effort and work of breathing. General exercise reconditioning can improve comfortable exercise tolerance and the retraining program can bring back *spring* once again.

Chapter IX

Oxygen

Oxygen is the breath of life. All tissues and cells must have oxygen for normal metabolism (see Chapter I). Certain tissues are more vulnerable than others to oxygen lack. For example, the brain can be without oxygen for only three to four minutes and the heart can be without oxygen for perhaps only thirty minutes before irreparable damage occurs. The dramatic effects of low oxygen on normal, healthy persons can best be exemplified by observations made upon athletes who ascend to high altitudes in mountain climbing expeditions. For example, when climbers ascend to more than 18,000 feet in climbing the Andes or Himalayas, the oxygen in the atmosphere and thus the inspired air becomes reduced by 50 per cent, and in spite of all efforts to eat energy-producing foods and maintain nutrition, a gradual progressive and massive weight-loss occurs. This is evidence of tissue breakdown from low oxygenation. Some patients with severe emphysema and chronic bronchitis, in similar fashion, can only provide a reduced oxygen supply to their tissues; in some of these patients, the oxygen-carrying capacity and thus the delivery of oxygen to the tissues is reduced by nearly 50 per cent. These patients also frequently lose weight and become wasted. As far as we know, this is due to lack of oxygenation of the tissues.

Oxygen has been available treatment for emphysema and chronic bronchitis for many years. It seems incredible that oxygen still remains a controversial therapy, in spite of large numbers of patients whose bodies literally plead for oxygen — the breath of life.

Oxygen was first discovered by an English Unitarian Minister, Joseph Priestley, in 1774. Priestley roasted chemicals called nitre and captured the escaping gas. He called his discovery dephlogisticated air, or pure air. Following considerable scientific investigation, Dr. Priestley and two mice eventually breathed the colorless gas and suffered no ill effects. Indeed, Priestley experienced a "light and easy" feeling which prompted him to declare "who can tell, but that in time this pure air may become a fashionable article in luxury." Oxygen may today be considered a luxury to some (scuba divers, high-altitude jumpers, and Alpine mountain climbers), but oxygen is the staff of existence for those who lack it and thus suffer from loss of the fuel which kindles the fire of life.

Actually, Priestley failed to appreciate the significance of his discovery. As always, in the annals of scientific medicine, no one advance stands by itself and it takes evaluation, re-evaluation, criticism, new interest, and wise people to recognize the value of discovery.

The fundamental principle of respiration was learned and enumerated by leaders of the day. Their names today are meaningless, but it hurts none of us to learn that Lavoisier, 1743-1794, first reported to doctors and nurses of the era the fundamental principles of respiration. Lavoisier knew that oxygen was consumed and that carbon dioxide, the product of the body's metabolism was exhaled. Lavoisier appreciated the fact that the lungs had to provide adequate oxygenation and carbon dioxide removal. Thus, by the end of the eighteenth century, the purpose of respiration had been discovered, and oxygen had been isolated. From that time onward, doctors devoted their attention toward further studies of respiration and how it may be deranged in disease.

Paul Bert worked in both low and high pressure chambers to simulate low and high altitudes. J. S. Haldane came to Colorado in 1909 to study the effects of the high altitude (14,110 ft.) of Pikes Peak on respiration.

One of the authors (Dr. Petty) spent two months doing high-altitude research atop Mt. Evans (14,260 feet) while a student of medicine. An anecdote from premedical years is included: "After carrying oxygen tanks across a snow field following the freshman year of medical training, I became exhausted and out of breath. It was difficult to sleep the first night in spite of a cot and a comfortable sleeping bag. Sleep was always difficult and at times I would awake, sit bolt upright in my sack and gasp for air; by morning I was tired, depressed, and had a terrible headache. It was necessary to abandon the experiment for two days while I retreated to a lower altitude to rest and to more oxygen."

I can remember the relief on descent from 14,000 feet to 5,000 feet. Today I appreciate this experience because I know what shortness of breath is, understand sleepless nights, and what terrible morning headaches can be. I have wished many times that the descent to a lower altitude would help my patients. It is usually not that simple. But later in this chapter we will show how oxygen therapy can be safely used in the home to the great benefit of the patient. It's better than taking your lungs to a lower altitude, for you can do it in your own home.

To finish the pre-med story, I returned to the laboratory at high altitude, adjusted to it, became interested in respiration and in lungs, as well as in patients with bad lungs. I'm glad!

Unfortunately, the hospital and particularly the home use of oxygen remains controversial in the minds of many because of certain ingrained fears concerning possible oxygen *toxicity*. Recent experience from our own laboratory has shown beyond question that oxygen at low concentrations is sufficient to bring blood oxygenation back to normal; oxygen is entirely safe when used properly. Oxygen is usually administered from a metal oxygen tank or from an oxygen source within a hospital. Tanks are also used in the home. Research has shown that low flows of oxygen such as a one to three liters per minute by an accurate flowmeter are sufficient to provide normal oxygenation. This flow increases the inspired oxygen concentration by 10 to 15 per cent and usually provides for normal oxygenation of the blood.

Oxygen is usually bubbled through water and then delivered through narrow conductive tubing to the patient's nose or mouth. Actually, bubbling oxygen through water adds very little water and the bubbling device can be avoided. Oxygen is usually administered via nasal prongs (Fig. 29) or with a variety of face masks. The nasal prongs allow the nose to provide its normal moisturizing function. Oxygen through the mouth is somewhat drying. We find that most patients tolerate nasal prongs very well and this method is now preferred by most experts. Several of our patients have continuously taken oxygen at home for several years with no adverse effects.

Oxygen is valuable in various situations. At rest, the body's needs for oxygen are least and we call this the *basal state*. When patients exercise, they need more oxygen to feed their muscles. Thus while enjoying increased activity, oxygen demands become greater. Patients with severe emphysema and bronchitis have to labor to breathe; therefore, the muscles of respiration require more oxygen for work. For this reason, oxygen is most useful during activity or when patients are having to labor to breathe because more oxygen is required for muscular activity and to pro-

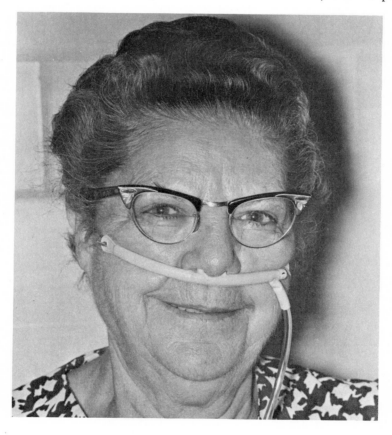

Figure 29. Oxygen delivered by double nasal prongs. Notice insertion into nares. This system is suitable for outpatient or inpatient oxygen delivery.

vide oxygen for the work of breathing. Patients may need oxygen for short periods such as ten to fifteen minutes following exertion necessary for daily living; oxygen inhalation may be helpful following a bath, while dressing, or during other forms of exertion.

We sometimes see patients who use oxygen only to power their breathing machines. It is our opinion that if patients exhibit a need for oxygen as proven by a low oxygen content of the blood, the need to supply oxygen to the tissues is always present, not just for periods of fifteen or twenty minutes. At any rate, during periods of deeper breathing with a machine, the blood oxygenation may be improved even with compressed air because of more breathing and thus more available oxygen in the lung.

We feel that because of the expense and difficulties involved in continuous oxygen therapy, many patients are denied this valuable drug. Patients can learn the safe use of home oxygen and, as with the use of any drugs, the proper dose must be used.

Prior to 1965, the policy at our hospital regarding the supply of continuous oxygen at home was up to the ingenuity of the doctor or patient involved. One of our patients has received continuous oxygen for nine years. She has suffered from severe tuberculosis of one lung and severe emphysema of the remaining lung. At first, physicians were reluctant to give this patient oxygen fearing that she would become addicted to it. (We would call to the attention of every reader of this book that we, too, are totally dependent or addicted to adequate oxygen in the tissues). We were finally able to begin continuous oxygen in the hospital with great improvement. As soon as oxygen was begun, the patient no longer labored to breathe in bed. We extended her care into the home and provided oxygen tanks for home use — this after many months in the hospital. From this point onward, the husband's ingenuity gained force. He built racks for carrying the oxygen tanks in the station wagon. He learned how to attach a smaller tank of oxygen to a wheeled carrier so that his wife could occasionally go outside into the yard to feel the sun and the breeze and to see the flowers.

Later, they went camping, taking all of the oxygen equipment with them. What wonderful recovery of life! It only took a little imagination on the part of the patient, her husband, and the physician along with the knowledge that continuous oxygen therapy was absolutely necessary and feasible for this particular patient.

To repeat, a certain number of patients have such inability to oxygenate the blood that they need oxygen at all times, both day and night. It is entirely safe to sleep with oxygen once the physician has learned what flow will provide normal oxygenation without dangerous effects. Oxygen must always be instituted and supervised by the patient's physician.

The main practical problem with continuous oxygen is its expense. *Continuous* oxygen costs from $150-$200 a month depending upon the type of oxygen used and the amount consumed. This is a very considerable expense for patients who are also burdened by large medical bills. However, when oxygen can be used to increase the patient's comfort and improve longevity, the expense seems reasonable. Furthermore, this therapy may prevent excessive hospitalization or the need for nursing home care. Certainly, oxygen is much less expensive than hospitalization or the nursing home.

Concern exists in the minds of many people about the possible fire hazard of oxygen therapy. It should be stressed that oxygen itself will not burn and is not explosive. Oxygen supports combustion; that is to say, it allows other things to burn. Oxygen should never be used near an open flame, and it goes without saying that patients should not smoke while they are using oxygen therapy. If smoking and open flames are not used in conjunction with oxygen, this gas, in the authors' opinion, becomes entirely safe for use in the home.

Oxygen should be used like any other drug, that is, under the supervision of a physician and in a controlled dose necessary to achieve the desired result. The goals of oxygen therapy are to provide oxygen for muscular activity, increased total activity, to lessen the work load on the heart, and to improve longevity.

We believe the only danger of home oxygen is "overdosage," and must stress that just like any other drug, oxygen has a safe level and a toxic level. Doctors are not afraid to give their diabetic patients insulin because of the possibility of insulin shock, but recognize the importance of patient education in the administration of this valuable pharmacological agent.

New advances have been made in oxygen therapy. Exceedingly simple and safe devices have been developed for home oxygen therapy. Industry has provided new means to deliver oxygen. This involves the use of excellent thermos bottle-like containers which are filled with very cold liquid oxygen. The container weighs only seven pounds and can easily be carried by a patient. The superb insulation of the container keeps the liquid oxygen cold and thus in the fluid state. Gradually, this liquid oxygen "boils" off into oxygen vapor which the patient breathes through a flow regulator connected to a tube, and from there to the two-pronged nasal cannula described earlier in this chapter.

This allows the patient mobility (Fig. 30). Our patient described earlier who has used conventional oxygen for nine years was recently provided with the new device. She told us a few months later that she went Christmas shopping alone for the first time in six years.

Fortunately the new devices called oxygen walkers are now generally available in most large cities in the United States. Problems in finding payments for these devices and in delivery in certain areas remain.

Simple compressed cylinders which can be filled from larger cylinders have been available for some years. Figure 31 shows such a device. These devices have a shorter supply of oxygen (usually 90 minutes) but are available to those who live away from large metropolitan centers where the liquid oxygen system is not available. We urge our patients to follow their physician's advice concerning home oxygen. One should not medicate himself with self-purchased oxygen. One should not rely on some of the other portable devices such as oxygen bulbs or canes. These only give a few whiffs of oxygen which can, at best, be of transient value. Home oxygen by conventional means and with ingenuity may bring great benefit and the new portable devices as well as further improvements already on the horizon will make oxygen therapy much easier and hopefully less expensive in the future.

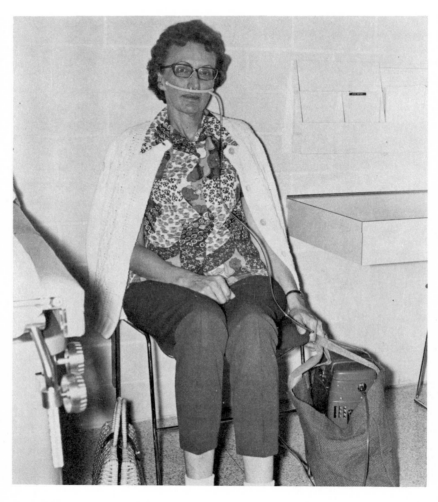

Figure 30. Patient with portable oxygen supply carried in handbag. This carries a 3 to 5-hour oxygen supply. Device can also be worn over shoulder using shoulder strap (Linde Oxygen Walker, New York, N.Y.).

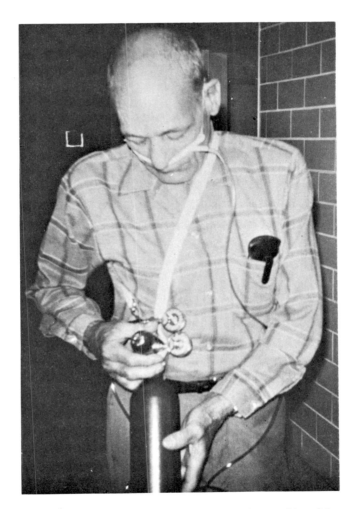

Figure 31. Small compressed oxygen bottle capable of being filled by larger oxygen cylinder (J.H. Emerson Company, Cambridge, Mass.).

Chapter X

Surgical Treatment

Mᴀɴʏ ꜱᴜʀɢɪᴄᴀʟ ᴏᴘᴇʀᴀᴛɪᴏɴꜱ ʜᴀᴠᴇ been devised to try and improve patients with chronic bronchitis and emphysema. Several of these operations have been studied in experimental animals and a number have been tried in human beings with less than dramatic results. This chapter is intended to review surgical treatment so that patients with emphysema and chronic bronchitis may be enlightened concerning possibilities and problems of surgical therapy.

Tracheostomy

Tracheostomy is a surgical opening in the windpipe or trachea (Fig. 32). This operation is highly beneficial and absolutely necessary in certain respiratory emergencies. The surgeon may perform a tracheostomy in the operating room, in the emergency room, or even in a patient's hospital bed. The operation can be performed safely and quickly with local Novocain® anesthesia. A tracheostomy has two basic purposes. First and most important is to provide an opening for removal of secretions when the patient cannot cough effectively. In this case, secretions are removed by means of a suction tube attached to a vacuum source. Secondly, a tracheostomy is used when *breathing machines* are needed to support life (Chapter VII). Tracheostomies are used primarily in acute situations where the secretion problem is progressing or when the need for a *ventilator* is critical. The mechanical removal of secretions and the use of mechanical ventilation are frequently life-saving measures. After the patient's recovery progresses to the point where a mechanical ventilator is no longer needed and the patient's own coughing efforts become strong enough to clear secretions, the tracheostomy tube is easily removed and the incision heals quite promptly, usually without a noticeable scar.

In a very few patients a permanent tracheostomy may be beneficial. Some patients have such a severe secretion problem and are so weak that they are unable to clear their lungs of mucus by coughing maneuvers. These few individuals are taught to suction themselves and to care for their tracheostomies at home. Patients must give their tracheostomies meticulous care in order to prevent infection occurring around the opening in the neck. Two *tracheostomy tubes* should be available, one for use and another clean tube for replacement. The tracheostomy tube should be changed at least twice a week to prevent accumulation of irritating mucus crusts. The skin opening should be cleansed with peroxide and cotton-tipped applicators every day or whenever crusts at the skin edge are found.

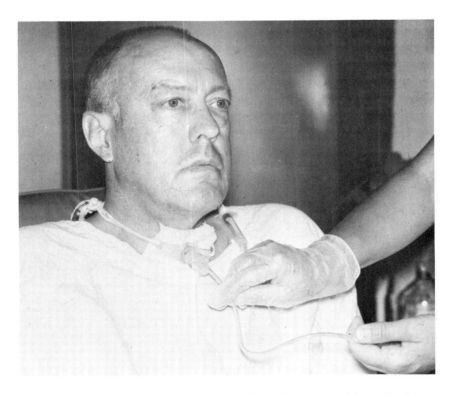

Figure 32. Technique of tracheostomy suction. The nurse with sterile-gloved hands, inserts a small plastic tube into the windpipe for purposes of suctioning secretions.

Dirty tracheostomy tubes should be washed in soap and water and scrubbed inside and out with a brush. For sterilization, soaking in Clorox® for ten minutes is effective, and Clorox will also whiten the plastic tracheostomy tube and thus avoid discoloration and staining.

We have not used a permanent tracheostomy for the past four years, because our experience has taught us that proper bronchial hygiene can be performed with proper use of home nebulizers, humidifiers, and breathing machines, when necessary, without resort to a permanent tracheostomy (Chapter VI).

We are pleased that we can now avoid permanent tracheostomies because of the potential of infection and also because we can avoid the problem of self-consciousness that some patients feel when in public with a tracheostomy.

We never advise removing a well-functioning tracheostomy if the patient has benefitted markedly from its use, for example in the case of a man we saw recently who had a permanent tracheostomy placed by a physician in another city. He had been desperately ill and simply unable to raise sputum. Numerous hospitalizations were necessary because of flare-ups of bronchitis caused, in part, by pooled secretions. After the tracheostomy was placed and secretions removed, a tremendous improvement was apparent immediately. Thus, this patient's physician decided to continue with the "trach" at home. We saw him six months later after a weight gain of fifty pounds, no more bouts of bronchitis and no more hospitalizations. We discussed the possibility of removal of the "trach" and using our method of bronchial hygiene, but we could detect immediate fear of removing something which had brought improvement and which now meant comfort and the ability to adjust to near-normal existence. Thus, our only criticism of the permanent tracheostomy is that infection may occur and that simpler means of proper bronchial hygiene are available.

Tracheal Fenestration

A tracheal fenestration is similar to a tracheostomy and is the so-called "window procedure." The surgeon forms skin flaps in the neck which are capable of being opened for the purpose of suctioning, but which close together when suctioning is not necessary. This allows the patient to have a permanent opening in his neck which is opened when it is needed for suctioning and closed when it is not needed. Patients with a fenestration can cough, strain, sneeze, and take IPPB treatments without air leaking through his neck in contrast to the tracheostomy patient who has air whistling through his neck during similar maneuvers. It is our opinion that fenestration may be beneficial in an occasional patient who cannot learn to cough and clear his lungs and who can be taught suctioning of secretions through the fenestration effectively at home. Fenestrations have the drawback of possible infection and slight disfigurement. We believe that it is far better if the patient can get by without a fenestration or a tracheostomy and can clear secretions by bronchial hygiene procedures (Chapter VI).

Carotid Body Denervation

A few surgeons in this country and abroad have tried a different and controversial approach to the treatment of emphysema and chronic bronchitis. Certain nerves pass from the brainstem where respiration and other vital functions are controlled (respiratory center) Chapter I, into the neck and from there to the so-called autonomic nerves attached to the airways. Some scientists once believed that nervous impulses traveling through these circuits may be important in the development of bronchospasm. For this reason, some surgeons have attempted to cut these nervous pathways in order to try and prevent bronchospasm. Whereas, literally thousands of these operations have been performed, studies on patients both before and after this procedure have failed to show any lasting benefit. It is our considered opinion that these denervation operations are of no value.

Carotid sinus denervation still has tremendous appeal in some sections of this country, primarily because this procedure represents "another hope" and patients are always looking for a simple and immediate method of therapy.

One of our patients asked us about this procedure and we did not recommend it. Although he learned and followed our program well, he ultimately had the operation in another city (cost for the operation alone was $500.00), but on his way home, he became seriously ill and stopped at our institution for further emergency care. After recovery, we repeated his breathing function tests (Chapter I) and found that he was, in fact, worse following the procedure. We do not believe the operation itself caused him to deteriorate. The point is that he definitely was not improved. The patient lives in another city, but we talked to his physician recently and received the report that the patient now can notice no improvement, only his banker could tell the difference!

Tracheal Support Operations

Since even the large airways including the trachea or windpipe collapse on expiration, some surgeons have devised operations to help support the airways. It is possible that these procedures may be beneficial in some patients. However, since all the airways throughout the lung collapse on expiration, it is unlikely that supporting simply the largest airway will be beneficial.

Surgical Removal of Lung

Occasionally there is a large area of emphysema which balloons out. These huge useless bubbles may compress the surrounding functioning lung. In these isolated and unusual situations, the removal of large destroyed bubbles, called *blebs* and *bullae,* may correct the situation and may allow the surrounding compressed lung to re-expand to its normal size and more efficiently participate in breathing. Patients should be studied very critically before surgery is contemplated in order to determine which patient may benefit from removal of these blebs and bullae.

Very rarely, removal of a whole diseased lobe may be profitable in order to allow remaining lobes to overexpand and be in a good position to breathe just a little more.

Except for tracheostomy which is an important and well-established procedure, and the fenestration operation which may be helpful in an occasional patient, it is our opinion that no surgical procedure has been proven effective in the treatment of emphysema or chronic bronchitis. We feel, however, that further surgical research should take place in order to determine whether any of the operations listed above or new operations can provide long-term improvement.

Finally, the budding era of transplantation gives us some new hopes for the future (Chapter XII). After further advances, it may be possible to transplant a lobe or a lung from a normal, healthy donor into the patient with severe emphysema and/or chronic bronchitis. This would be similar to the more established procedure of kidney transplantation. Enormous scientific and technical problems remain and, at the present time, lung transplantation is not being performed except rarely and in the experimental animal. This procedure may be very important in the future.

Chapter XI

Daily Living

Many patients with chronic bronchitis and emphysema become discouraged concerning their plight and feel that much of what is important and pleasant in life must be abandoned in order to protect themselves against the progress of their disease. This attitude is wrong and leads to a feeling of hopelessness and loss of interest in what is precious and dear concerning life. It also causes a growing concern about oneself that can damage one's emotional structure and interfere with treatment.

An attitude of despair actually leads to abandonment of the very things which can bring lasting benefit. If one loses interest in breathing training and physical reconditioning, if the bronchial hygiene program falls by the wayside, and if the prescribed medications are not utilized, quite naturally any earlier benefit may be lost and deterioration may occur. There is another side to this problem. Some patients become so ritualistic with the medical and rehabilitation program that they abandon normal living activities. This attitude is equally wrong.

This chapter is designed to re-emphasize the importance of adjustment to the limitation of one's illness but still being active and hopefully leading a normal life. This is an important chapter.

The Daily Routine

Medical treatment, bronchial hygiene, and the physical reconditioning program must be worked into the daily routine. Life should not be curtailed by the need to follow a somewhat complex program. Indeed, the whole purpose of pulmonary rehabilitation, which is really our ultimate goal, in the care of emphysema and chronic bronchitis, is to provide the health and stamina for daily living. So our prescription for rehabilitation must not interfere with fun, adventure, or happiness.

Some of the following repeats material presented in earlier chapters. Our aim is to explain how a well-conceived and coordinated medical and rehabilitation program is compatible with daily living.

On arising each morning, the bronchial hygiene prescription should be followed. During sleep, mucus collects and thus the morning treatment period is most necessary and is apt to be most productive. First, the patient will nebulize inhaled bronchodilator for four to five minutes to achieve maximum airway decongestion. This is followed by the inhalation of warm or cold moisture for ten to fifteen minutes and then either controlled coughing efforts or postural drainage can be utilized to remove the accumulated mucus. This procedure should take no more than twenty-five to thirty minutes. Medication which is given once a day, such as digitalis, should be taken at this point as well as the morning dose of any drug which is given three times daily (e.g., the oral bronchodilator). After personal hygiene, dressing and breakfast, one may rest, read the morning paper, or walk around the house or yard a bit, perhaps not being too active in order to allow for digestion, and in some patients to allow for the increase in shortness of breath which may follow full meals. One should eat a full breakfast.

After this brief rest, the morning exercise program should be instituted. Each patient should plan to be a bit more active. Walk to the next tree, visit the neighbor down the block or utilize your best time of day (often the morning) for doing necessary tasks such as grocery shopping. If sudden shortness of breath occurs during this period, use the metered-dose pocket device for two or three breaths if away from home or the powered or hand bulb nebulizer at home.

Before lunch, take noontime medication such as the oral bronchodilator and have a leisurely lunch to promote the maximum intake of nutritious food, especially if underweight. An afternoon nap is refreshing and beneficial. On awakening, a short period of nebulization, steaming, and clearing mucus may or may not be needed. Another walk is needed in midafternoon. One need not simply walk for walking's sake — a visit to the museum or art gallery or to the park or zoo may cover many yards or miles of walking. Be sure to concentrate on breathing. If tightness or wheeze occur, use the metered bronchodilator once or twice again.

The evening meal should not be a large one. This is the least necessary meal of the day because after a short while sleep will follow. This is the daily period of least activity. It is a little better to take the third dose of a medication taken three times daily with supper than at bedtime because some bronchodilators may tend to interfere with sleep.

After supper, another shorter stroll may make one sleepy and ready for bed. The bronchial hygiene program of bronchodilator, moisture, and expulsive coughing should be performed at bedtime to prepare one for sleep. Sedatives for routine use are not safe and actually sedatives are rarely needed for sleep. The daily routine and the relaxation gained through physical reconditioning will often allow patients to obtain more restful sleep than at any other time in recent years. When sleep does not come immediately, reading will usually tire the eyes and sleep will come.

Most patients appreciate the flow of fresh air into the bedroom. While the bedroom should not be excessively cool, one should not fear some fresh air. Colds are caused by a virus and not by a normal amount of fresh air.

Occasionally, patients will awaken at night with some accumulated mucus. Often a moderate cough or a simple throat clearing will remove the secretions. If marked tightness is present, use of the hand bulb or powered nebulizer will help stop a bout of bronchospasm. If one becomes fully awakened by the need to nebulize, it is often well to eat a snack such as milk and crackers or read awhile until the urge to sleep returns.

We have described an average program which will work better for some than others. We stress flexibility. Certainly life's patterns should not become rigid. Some people are more active at night than during the daytime. One may spend the evening at a party and then prefer to sleep late. Our principle remains regular bronchial hygiene on arising and retiring and at least two daily graded exercise periods and always proper breathing. Of course, the total program is suitable for one at work. This patient may well get his exercise while at work.

The above regimen may not work at first. Remember, the disability of emphysema and chronic bronchitis has been long developing. One may take days or weeks to develop a simple scheme applying the above principles. But the principles are sound and eventually will work.

Many of our patients come to us with other questions concerning certain habits, diet, and many other problems. The following portion of the chapter will give advice concerning some of the most frequently asked questions.

Place of Residence

Extremes of high altitude are harmful because the oxygen concentration in the air decreases with altitude. At Denver, the mile-high city at 5,200 feet, the concentration of oxygen in the atmosphere is reduced by 13 per cent. This is not terribly burdensome, but at higher altitudes such as 8,000 to 10,000 feet, the burden of low oxygen in the atmosphere makes residence at these altitudes undesirable. Should everyone with chronic bronchitis or emphysema go to sea level? This question is frequently asked. Whereas there is some advantage in going from very high altitude such as greater than 6,000 to 7,000 feet down to sea level, very little advantage is gained in those patients living at 2,000 to 3,000 feet in descent to a slightly lower altitude. Balance this slight gain against leaving ones friends, family, and a familiar environment, and it usually is not desirable for a patient to pick up all of his belongings and travel to a distant city simply to achieve low altitude. When family ties are not strong and in those patients with "wanderlust" it may be valuable to take a trip to a low altitude and see how one feels in the new environment. The Tuscon, Phoenix, and southern California areas have become tremendously popular for patients with chronic lung disease. Perhaps low altitudes coupled by bright sunshine, freedom from cold temperature as well as the fraternal spirit of living among those who have learned to adjust to life with chronic bronchitis and emphysema in the warm, dry climate of the southwest is of value. Others may dislike the association of similarly afflicted individuals and find large groups of emphysema or bronchitis patients depressing. Most patients who are recovering from their disease, however, are not depressed.

Perhaps in certain cases, these advantages are worth a move.

But in our experience even at the altitude of Denver, Colorado, patients with severe lung disease can learn to adjust to their environment. At times, additional oxygen therapy is needed for comfortable existence or for the accomplishment of the exercise program, but this can be provided (Chapter IX).

A number of our cities are becoming progresisvely polluted with automobile exhaust, industrial emissions, and other sources of air pollution and it is probably undesirable to continue to live in a very heavily polluted area, everything else considered. When possible, it is wise not only to avoid the irritant of smoking, but also the irritation of prolonged exposure to heavily polluted air. It must be stressed, however, that the vast majority of cities in this country do not have the degree of air polution that is particularly damaging to the lung. Again the rule of living where one is happiest should be followed. We do not advise moving away from cities of moderate air pollution unless there is no particular reason to remain.

Diet

No particular food is harmful to emphysema patients. One problem with emphysema patients is that they frequently become short of breath while eating and consequently eat less food and lose weight. This may interfere with maintenance of muscular strength. It is important then to eat frequent small meals such as five to six a day including snacks between meals occasionally. Small meals will tend to avoid gaseous overdistention which some patients experience. We try to avoid obesity, but it is clear that a good state of nutrition is an important health measure which will allow patients with emphysema and chronic bronchitis to be active longer and perhaps to feel better. When fluid retention occurs in associated heart failure, salt restriction is needed but this isn't necessary in the average case.

In addition, it should be stressed that patients with emphysema and chronic bronchitis have an increased incidence of *peptic ulcer* disease. The reason for this is entirely unknown, but the observations have been clearly established in many centers. Thus, again it is important for patients to eat nutritious food frequently, and it is undoubtedly important to eat often so as to have food in the stomach in order to avoid excessive gastric acidity and thus the peptic ulceration.

Sleep

Earlier chapters describing medical treatment, surgical treatment, bronchial hygiene, and exercise have stressed a rather aggressive onslaught against the disease on the part of both the patient and his physician in an attempt to curb the progress of emphysema and chronic bronchitis. Our ultimate aim is to develop a rehabilitation program which will lead to freedom from distressing symptoms, provide for increased activity, and probably increased longevity. Thus, it is important for our patients not only to work hard for their rehabilitation program, but also to have pauses for rest and sleep which are important. Quiet relaxing sleep is beneficial to any patient. Whereas we advise no special prescription for sleep, the usual seven to eight hours are the basic minimum and additional rest periods and naps are important. Sleep can be programmed into the overall rehabilitation program. Very often an evening walk followed by a small snack will render the patient quite sleepy and ready for rest. On awakening the next morning, hopefully fully rested, an increased exercise program is often possible. Thus sleep is important in all facets of the patient's rehabilitation. It should be stressed that sleeping pills and tranquilizers are not generally advisable because these drugs may dangerously depress respiration during sleep. An evening nightcap such as one to two ounces of whiskey, a glass of wine, or a glass of beer may be all the sedation that is needed. Furthermore, when breathing retraining is learned, and exercise program followed, diet satisfactory, usually sleep-inducing medications are no longer needed.

The importance of exercise in the overall rehabilitation program has been amply stressed in Chapter VIII. Exercise should be stressed again as exceedingly important to the rehabilitation measures and one should recall that the ability to exercise provides for the resumption of normal daily activities, often abandoned by emphysema patients.

Alcohol

Alcohol in moderate quantities is not harmful to the lungs. Research indicates that alcohol is excreted through the lungs to a certain extent, and if large amounts of alcohol continually pass through the lungs, irritation is possible. Also the patient who consumes large quantities of alcohol frequently also smokes cigarettes; this is a double hazard to the lungs. It remains our opinion that the cocktail or two before dinner, wine with dinner, or an occasional beer is not harmful. As a matter of fact, alcohol, one of the world's oldest and safest drugs if used properly, is probably the safest and most beneficial tranquilizing agent for patients with emphysema and chronic bronchitis.

Sex

It has been our observation in many of our patients that when emphysema and chronic bronchitis become severe, sexual activity is greatly curtailed. Men with these diseases indicate lack of interest and a definite development of impotence occurs. Females become particularly uninterested in sex. The reasons for this are not entirely known; however, the presence of continued shortness of breath, the fears and anxieties concerning the chronic illness, and the feeling present on both the part of patients and physicians that life is hopeless, life is useless, and thus life must be curtailed, lead to an emotional loss of normal sex interest.

We have learned, in contrast, that as patients improve through bronchial hygiene, breathing exercises, and the overall rehabilitation program, as patients understand their disease and know that life is no longer hopeless that increased sexual awareness and ability returns. We believe this is part of an emotional readjustment to an underlying disease. As patients become able to exercise in the graded exercise program (Chapter VIII), so can they also tolerate the increased activity of normal sexual intercourse.

As a final comment to this chapter, we should stress that the development of emphysema and chronic bronchitis is at least as disabling from emotional factors as it is from physical factors. Curtailing all of life's precious activities should not be the goal of the emphysema patient. A patient of the author's comes to mind at this point.

We recently saw a man who was desperately ill and wasted from the ravages of long-standing emphysema. On review of his life's history, it was apparent that two years ago he entered a nursing home in order to simplify his life. In the nursing home, he lost interest in all normal activity and simply vegetated, spending most of his time in bed. But when admitted to our hospital with a final illness, the following question was asked "You have not been to the clinic or hospital for two years. What have you been doing in the nursing home?" The answer was a pitiful reply. "I've been breathing, just breathing." This sorry resume of the past two years of "life" is the epitome of what we are trying to avoid by writing this book. It is obvious that this poor patient abandoned all of life in order to try and protect himself. In doing so, he also abandoned every chance for survival or rehabilitation because he simply gave up his interest, gave up enthusiasm for life and thus lost every opportunity to participate in the programs of education, self-care, and rehabilitation which are subjects of earlier chapters. If this attitude can be avoided by even a few patients who read this book, another of our major objectives will have been realized.

Chapter XII

The Outlook Today and the Future

THE PRECEDING ELEVEN CHAPTERS have been an effort on the part of a chest physician and a respiratory care nurse to explain, hopefully in simple language, what is known about chronic bronchitis and emphysema, what can be done today in terms of specific treatment, and what can be done in the area of rehabilitation. The preceding chapters have given simple but current and factual information concerning the management of emphysema and chronic bronchitis. In the light of what has been presented before and in the light of modern-day knowledge, what is the outlook for emphysema and chronic bronchitis patients today? What do we envision in the future?

For severe cases where irreparable lung damage has taken place, the outlook must be one of guarded enthusiasm. In the case of respiratory failure when lungs are not providing enough oxygenation to support life, we have the know-how to gain time with the use of superb breathing machines. If our therapeutic efforts are successful, we can look forward to the recovery of perhaps 60 to 80 per cent of these cases depending on the underlying condition. We know that even these patients can be rehabilitated and can live happy and healthy years in spite of the serious medical emergency. Some patients can return to work. Respiratory care centers are being developed in many cities to provide modern medical and nursing care in intensive respiratory care units. These centers provide excellent equipment along with expert technical ability. By use of this available equipment, better care is realized today.

We have observed a curious phenomenon in many patients who recover from acute respiratory failure. A few weeks after leaving the hospital, these patients often tell us that they feel and breathe better than at any time in recent years. How can they feel improved after a life threatening bout of respiratory failure? The answer may lie in the fact that during the episode of respiratory failure, we have cleared the airways better than they have ever been cleared before by suction through a tracheostomy. This may well have been the beginning of good bronchial hygiene, which then was continued after discharge from the hospital. Additional reasons for the newly felt awareness of well-being understandably come from the benefits of breathing retraining and general physical reconditioning. A further factor may be the knowledge that the lung condition has not been hopeless after all, and that with the recovery experienced, that "new lease on life feeling" explains some of the exhilaration demonstrated by these patients.

If our reasoning that a good medical and physical program has really improved patients to this degree, it seems a pity that the patient must suffer an episode of life-threatening respiratory failure in order to get better. Actually with conviction and enthusiasm applied to other less seriously ill patients, the same improvement is often appreciated.

For the patient with moderate shortness of breath and only mild or moderate limitation, the outlook is really quite bright. If our educational programs to curtail smoking and avoid the excessive irritation of air pollution in certain cities are successful, if patients can learn to understand their disease, alert their physicians when infections are only beginning, and participate in a well-organized home-care program, we believe that the progress of disease can often be stopped and patients can live a fully normal life with their remaining breathing function. We have some evidence which shows that healing of the bronchitis portion of the disease may take place. One patient of ours who was in severe respiratory failure and whose life was being supported by a ventilator nearly two years ago made a complete recovery. He is the patient cited earlier who works full time as a filling station attendant at an altitude of 8,000 feet and claims that he has absolutely no shortness of breath. It has been interesting to note that in our laboratory we find his pulmonary function is reduced by only 50 per cent. This is like having only one lung after surgical removal of the other. We compare this patient to the many patients living comfortable lives with only one lung. This patient's pulmonary function has not deteriorated over the last two years.

This is because he has stopped smoking. We have reason to believe that further deterioration will not take place and we have every hope that a near normal life expectancy will be realized. However, the dramatic improvement in this case was made possible not only by virtue of excellent methods of medical management and nursing care, but also because the patient was willing to learn about his disease, was willing to stop smoking, and was willing to participate in an excellent home-care program as outlined by many of the earlier chapters of this book.

One of the greatest advances in the care and rehabilitation of disabled patients has been the knowledge that continuous oxygen can be safely given and furthermore that continuous oxygen is often effective in reducing the extra burden on the heart which frequently occurs in emphysema and chronic bronchitis. Continuous oxygen is equally effective in controlling the excessive blood formation which occurs in patients who have impaired oxygenation of their blood.

Going hand in hand with the scientific research which has proven the value of continuous oxygen has been the development of portable oxygen equipment to allow patients to be active, do more, and live normal lives. The impact of continuous oxygen on an individual case may be tremendous.

A number of our patients have received continuous ambulatory oxygen for periods exceeding five years. In some cases, they have been able to return to work and participate in gainful employment for extended periods. One of our earliest patients, with sixty-seven days of hospitalization prior to oxygen, has had only three days of hospitalization subsequently, encompassing a five-year period. His disease process remains extremely stable. Oxygen is most beneficial for those who are the most deficient in oxygen. We recognize that oxygen lack occurs more commonly at high altitudes than at lower altitudes. On the other hand, approximately one half of the inhabitable United States exists at the *modest* altitude of Denver and so this is not an unusual altitude. Oxygen is most valuable in patients that suffer heart failure related to lung problems (cor pulmonale). At the time of the writing of this second edition, oxygen is available by the liquid system in most metropolitan centers and by simple compressed gas systems elsewhere in the United States. Its physiological benefits has been established.

Other bright factors in the overall picture is the availability of potent antibiotics to treat infections and the development of many excellent pieces of equipment for bronchial hygiene.

The overall outlook may be exceedingly bright or exceedingly grim to a large number of patients who are really quite healthy today. This may be the smoker with the morning cough, but no other symptoms, or the young business executive who prefers to take the golf cart rather than exercise because of shortness of breath. This group includes the secretary who gives up hiking on weekends and instead sits and smokes in admiration of her television set, or a housewife who wants a one-story house because climbing stairs causes shortness of breath — others in this class may be the minister who gives his sermons in short sentences or the teenager who is just beginning to cough and produce sputum when he or she coughs.

Within this large heterogenous group, we often have an individual with early disease and little destruction. This is the situation where we can often stop disease in its tracks, prevent progression, and hopefully provide for normal life expectancy. We have the greatest hopes and yet the greatest fears for this type of patient. Our hopes are based upon the fact that irreversible lung deterioration is not present and therapeutic measures should be successful to promote healing of airway irritation, but our fears are based upon the complacency of human nature. It is very difficult at times to convince such patients that curtailment of smoking, participation in physical medicine procedures, and the adherence to detailed medical advice at this juncture are important. Why do patients wait until they are desperately ill before seeking medical advice? This is a question for psychiatrists, psychologists and sociologists to consider. This complacency may be the underlying factor leading to chronic disease in many cases. Whereas we should be able to help the mild case, we all too often are not allowed even to try!

Today, in this country we have at least fourteen million patients with chronic bronchites and emphysema. Emphysema deaths probably number 100,000. This is just as many deaths as result from lung cancer or from automobile accidents combined. Perhaps the true number, if all patients were discovered, would be twice or four times as great.

Emphysema and chronic bronchitis together are second only to heart disease as medical ailments requiring Social Security Disability. Many patients with chronic bronchitis and emphysema, we believe, are actually included in the heart disease group. We are probably only viewing the "visible part of an iceberg" in the overall problem.

The future promises additional advances. New breathing machines are on the horizon both for simplified home-care and for use in the hospital intensive care unit where respiratory failure is being managed. We have been involved in the evaluation and development of several devices which are now marketed.

These and other devices are making home care much more simple and practical. As expressed in early chapters, self-care is important in chronic disease. We are convinced that most patients do not need the assistance of medical or allied health personnel to provide their necessary bronchial hygiene techniques at home (see Chapter VI).

Concerning smoking, industry is trying its best to find a "safe cigarette." Since knowledge concerning the risks of smoking cigarettes has taken years to become evident, the authors would not trust any "safe cigarette" until it had been tested for at least twenty years. Our biggest hope for the future is the development of smoking clinics at various centers in this country. The approach of the successful Alcoholics Anonymous is the approach that should be copied. With education and group therapy, perhaps an increasing number of patients can be encouraged or taught to stop smoking.

Rehabilitation programs are being implemented in various centers in the country. Thus, in the future, the medical public will have somewhere to go for an organized rehabilitation program. The authors feel, however, that all physicians are in the position to provide and supervise a good pulmonary rehabilitation program. This fact should be obvious to anyone who has read this book. Details of bronchial hygiene and physical reconditioning can easily be practiced in the home. Our interest in the rehabilitation center is to have a training place for physicians, nurses, and technicians so that additional medical personnel can gain the know-how necessary to provide sophisticated care.

The possibilities of lung transplantation remain for the future. Certainly lung transplantation as mentioned in Chapter X is technically feasible, and our colleagues have already transplanted lungs or lobes of lungs from one experimental animal to another. Thus, the surgeon already has the know-how. The problems in lung transplantation have remained essentially three. First a suitable donor may be difficult to find since removal of a whole lung may somewhat disable the donor. However, even a lobe which could more easily be given up may be beneficial. Research must learn methods of organ storage. If, when natural death occurs, lungs can be saved for a later transplantation, the donor problem will be largely solved. The second problem with all organ transplantations is the high risk of infection. Even in kidney transplantation, which is reasonably successful, the necessity of interferring with body's defense mechanisms which tend to destroy the transplanted organ have lead to the serious problem of a variety of bacterial, fungus, parasitic and viral infections of the lung which are not generally amenable to antibiotic therapy. When more acceptable methods to prevent organ rejection are available and when more effective antibiotics to combat troublesome infection are found, then perhaps the infection problem will not be as serious. Certainly a transplantation, if successful, could benefit many patients. We believe the third problem with lung transplantation has been solved; that is means of effective ventilatory support of patients in the period after the operation. We believe that our new breathing machines will effectively support the patient of the future who may successfully have a lung transplantation.

Of course, new drugs may become available which will more effectively thin mucus and will replace our current bronchodilators. Other drugs may help unburden the heart in patients with severe lung disease.

We already know that the company making the liquid oxygen systems is working on a new device which will weigh less than 50 per cent of the original device (now approximately seven pounds) and which will carry even more oxygen. We believe this will replace the already excellent oxygen walkers in the future.

Research is beginning to increase our understanding of lung defense mechanisms. Questions concerning why some patients' lungs are damaged by cigarette smoking and air pollution and others are not very likely have to do with the ability of the lung to adapt or defend itself against irritation. This has been discussed in earlier chapters. Already one factor, the alpha antitrypsin deficiency state, a long chemical term for hereditary weakness in the ability of the lung to combat inflammation, has been fairly well ellucidated in the past five years. In addition, defects in immune responses have also been identified. If scientists can develop a series of relatively simple and practical tests for the identification of patients whose lung defenses are not what they should be, perhaps biochemical control and the alteration of risk factors such as smoking, infections and allergic problems could take on increased importance. Genetic counseling may be important in those identified as having potential or partial problems in pulmonary defenses. We are convinced that medical research will identify further factors which explain why emphysema and chronic bronchitis occur in certain patients and not in others and hopefully physicians will be able to capitalize on new knowledge in efforts to stem the tide of progressive disease.

Let us conclude this book which we have written for patients and have devoted to improvement of patient care and to pulmonary rehabilitation. Modern day medical science has given us excellent tools for the care of patients with emphysema and chronic bronchitis. We and colleagues throughout the country estimate that 80 to 85 per cent of the patients with these two diseases can be benefitted. Those with mildest degrees of disease can be benefitted perhaps the most, and yet even the most severe cases including those whose life must be supported for a time by breathing machines can be improved. Modern medical research continues and advances will be made in the future, but today we already have a massive armamentarium capable of altering the course of these two diseases if only they were applied. If the researcher over the next ten years made no new advances, still our patients could improve with use of existing knowledge. For this reason, it is important for patients and physicians alike to realize that with emphysema and chronic bronchitis, we do not face a helpless scourge, but rather two closely related diseases that are better understood than ever before and for which today we have effective treatment.

Glossary

aerosolize: The act of nebulizing medications for inhalation into the lungs.

air hunger: The sensation of insufficient oxygen or insufficient breathing.

air pollution: This term refers to grossly polluted air in our cities. The air pollution consists of hydrocarbons from automobile exhaust and oxides of nitrogen and sulfur. Whereas the dusty air of the plains is impressive, the inhalation of this ground dust is probably not harmful to the lungs. Also, people in various industries which are mildly dusty wonder about the association of the inhalation of these dusts. Dry cheese dust, for example, is not harmful. Most individuals who feel irritation while at work are actually heavy smokers and fail to realize that their cough and expectoration is coming from the old troublesome smoking habit.

allergy: Abnormal reaction to a stimulus called an allergen. In the context of this book, allergy refers to the abnormal response of the airways to inhaled stimuli such as pollen or to consumed items such as foods which may cause unusual airway reaction leading to the phenomenon of bronchospasm.

alveoli: Sac-like structures at the end of the conducting airways for the exchange of oxygen and carbon dioxide.

antibiotic: A drug which kills or inhibits bacteria. Whereas antibiotics are exceedingly effective in deep chest infections where bacterial invasion is almost always present, it should be stressed that antibiotics do not prevent the common cold and will not stop a cold that has developed. These drugs are simply effective against the bacterial invaders which follow the original cold virus.

autonomic nerves: Nerves that control organ function; so-called visceral nerves. Nervous impulses may alter organ function including the lungs.

bacteria: Infectious organisms which may produce bronchitis or pneumonia.

basal state: State of minimum metabolism where oxygen requirements are least.

black pigment: That which gives the damaged human lung the black and sooty appearance. The exact identity of the pigment has never been determined. It is related to cigarette smoking and to urban living. It is always found in emphysema and bronchitis. Whether the pigment is involved in the disease process is not known.

blebs and bullae: Localized destroyed portions of the lung which may occupy large portions of the thorax and occasionally compress otherwise useful lungs.

blood gas determinations: The direct measurement of oxygen and carbon dioxide in the blood. To accurately determine the blood gases, the physician samples arterial blood directly from an artery. This must be done because only blood which has circulated through the lungs will tell the true oxygen content.

booster: A single shot of a vacine designed to reawaken the protective response following original immunization.

breath sounds: Heard by the physician's stethoscope; the intensity of the sound of air moving in and out of the lungs gives an indication of the amount of obstruction.

breathing machine: A device which can support or control breathing; also called a ventilator. (These are fully discussed in Chapter VII.)

bronchial hygiene: In brief, it is a method to cleanse the lungs and airways of irritants and retained secretions. It is the act of inhaling a bronchodilator, followed by steam, followed by expulsive coughing efforts to clear the airway with or without postural drainage maneuvers to facilitate the drainage of secretions.

bronchodilator therapy: The use of drugs which combat musculature spasm of the conducting airways and helps to enlarge the constricted airways.

bronchospasm: A sudden narrowing of the airways due in part to contraction of the circular musculature of the conducting airways, in part to inflammatory swelling of the airway lining, and in part to secretions in the airways.

bronchus: The two main divisions of the trachea, one for each lung. These in turn branch some twenty times before the gas exchange membrane is reached.

capillaries: The smallest of blood vessels which also provide for the exchange of oxygen and carbon dioxide in the lungs. The small capillary branches join into large vessels to carry oxygenated blood to the tissues.

cartilage: (gristle) A ridged, yet flexible supporting tissue, somewhat similar in structure to bone but without bone's rigidity.

catarrh: The excessive production of mucus associated with a mild chronic cough. This chronic cough and expectoration probably signifies chronic bronchitis.

chronic obstructive lung disease: A broad encompassing term which includes emphysema, chronic bronchitis, and chronic asthma. Physicians sometimes like to use this somewhat noncommittal term because it admits the fact that elements of all three major diseases may be present in a given patient. The term chronic airway obstruction is also used for the same purpose. There will probably be more such nonspecific terms until scientists settle on specific criteria for the diagnosis of emphysema, chronic bronchitis, and chronic asthma.

cilia: The hairlike structures which line the airways and beat rhythmically away from the lungs in order to propel the mucous blanket toward the mouth. The cilia are a major cleansing mechanism of the lung.

cor-pulmonale: Strain of the right heart in emphysema and chronic broncihtis.

cortisone drugs: A family of steroid compounds that are anti-inflammatory. This includes prednisone (Meticortin® and other names) as well as a variety of related drugs.

cupped hands: Placing the hands into a position as to be able to hold water. The hands are then turned downward in a pounding and "cupping" percussion of the lungs.

decongestion: The reduction of swelling of nasal passages by nose drops. These function in a manner similar to inhaled bronchodilators.

diuretics: A group of drugs which promote kidney's excretion of salt and water (Diuril®, HydroDIURIL®, Esidrix®, and a variety of others). No effective diuretic is presently sold over the counter.

dyspnea: The medical term referring to shortness of breath. Literally, dyspnea means "bad breath" and physicians and patients alike agree that it is bad when one can't get one's breath.

edema: Swelling of the extremities due to salt and water retention. Some patients recognize edema themselves by tight shoes and tight stockings. Squeezing on edematous legs leaves an imprint of the thumb or fingers.

effluent: Streaming outward from any system such as moisture from a nebulizer.

elastic superstructure: Interwoven stretchable fibers which surround the alveoli and conducting airways and aid in inspiration and expiration.

electrocardiogram: A tracing of the heart's electrical activity; an important indicator of heart strain and other heart diseases. The electrocardiograph records the heart's activity, sensing tiny electrical impulses from the heart. The test utilizes electrodes strapped to the arms, legs, and chest.

expectorant: A drug which professes to improve the thinning and removal of secretions. The effectiveness of the various expectorants is open to great debate.

expiration: The release of stale air from the lungs; the act of breathing out.

fenestrations: Holes in the alveolar walls. Scientists believe that fenestrations are the first evidence of damaged alveolar walls, the essence of emphysema.

genetic: Refers to heredity; one possible cause of emphysema and possibly bronchitis.

heart failure: The inability of the heart to meet its work load. When the heart is strained, its output of blood is diminished and thus the kidneys do not receive sufficient circulation to excrete a normal quantity of salt and water. The term heart failure does not imply that the heart is hopelessly damaged, but that the heart is temporarily not doing enough work. Heart failure can be treated with drugs to stimulate the heart (digitalis) and even more importantly, treatment of the lung condition will often unburden the heart.

humidification: The act of moisturization.

inflammation: The process of irritation, reddening, and swelling of tissues.

inspiration: The taking of air into the lungs.

irritant: Any noxious substance which may damage the lungs.

life: That for which living is designed.

lobeline: A drug similar to nicotine in its affect on body function.

lymph glands: Pea-sized glands containing lymphatic cells. These glands are an important defense mechanism against infection and also are the stations in which irritants such as tar are deposited by the scavenger cells (macrophages).

lymphatic channels: Delicate vessels which carry the flow of a clear fluid (lymph) to the lymph glands.

macrophage: The scavenger cells of the lung which have the ability to consume and carry away lung irritants.

medulla: The most primitive portion of the brain which contains the centers of vital organ functions, such as the respiratory center.

metabolism: The consumption of oxygen and nutrients for energy production and for the maintenance of body tissues.

mucolytic agent: The term "lytic" refers to the ability to dissolve something. Thus, it is implied in the term "mucolytic" that we have drugs that can dissolve mucus. Whereas this is partly true, we still do not have the ideal drug to thin secretions. Numerous drugs will perform this task; they are somewhat irritating but still useful.

mucous glands: The glands that normally provide mucus for the cleansing of the lungs. These glands are enlarged in chronic bronchitis.

nebulizer: A device which breaks liquid into tiny droplets of suitable size for inhalation into the lungs.

now: Immediately, not tomorrow!

oxygen transport: The delivery of oxygen to the tissues. The term implies normal oxygenation of the blood and the delivery of this oxygenated blood to all the tissues of the body, a function of circulation.

panacea: A term referring to a "cure all." Unfortunately, there aren't any.

particle size: Refers to the size of the nebulized droplets of moisture or bronchodilator. Large particles deposit on the larger airways and smaller particles deposit on the finer airways of the lungs.

pedometer: A device which measures distance in walking. It appears similar to a watch and functions by pendulum action to record distance travelled.

phlebotomy: The therapeutic withdrawal of blood; usually a pint is removed.

physiologic: Referring to body function (normal or abnormal).

pleura: The delicate thin membrane which encases the lungs and lines the chest cavity.

pneumonia: A sudden infection of localized areas of the lungs; episodes of pneumonia frequently accompany bronchitis.

postural drainage: The act of positioning oneself in certain postures so as to allow gravity to help drain the lungs (Figs. 21, 22, 23, and 24).

prophylactic treatment: The term "prophylaxis" refers to prevention and the so-called prophylactic antibiotic treatment implies the possibility of preventing infection.

protuberant: The act of allowing the abdomen to pouch outward during inspiration.

red blood cells: The cells which give the blood its red color; also the cells which contain hemoglobin and carry oxygen to the tissues.

resistance: In the context of this book, resistance refers to impediment to air flow in and out of the lungs.

respirable size particles: Those smaller particles which can be inhaled deep into the lungs.

respiration: Not only the act of taking air into the lungs, but the act of delivering oxygen to the tissues and returning carbon dioxide to the lungs for removal.

respiratory center: An area in the brain which controls respiration; the respiratory center is stimulated by oxygen lack and excessive carbon dioxide as well as muscular activity.

respiratory failure: The sudden situation in which the lungs are not providing normal oxygenation or normal carbon dioxide removal.

sedative: A drug designed to promote sleep. These are dangerous in chronic lung disease.

side effects: Undesirable reactions to drugs. In the case of the steroid drugs, one finds a swelling of the face, salt and water retention, irritation to the stomach occasionally leading to ulcers, and a variety of less common but severe reactions.

somnolence: Excessive sleepiness. May occur from drugs or from severe states of respiratory failure where the lungs are not providing adequate oxygenation and carbon dioxide removal.

spirometer: A machine which measures breathing capacity. This may be a simple hand-held device which roughly estimates breathing capacity or may be a more complicated device which appears to be something akin to a large tin can which travels up and down with each breath.

sputum: Expectorated mucus or phlegm.

stethoscope: The ear piece that physicians use to examine the heart and lungs.

suppository: A preparation of drugs for placement into the rectum. Following insertion, the outer waxy covering dissolves allowing the drug to be absorbed into the lining of the rectum.

tenacious: A term referring to thick stringy, and difficult to remove secretions.

thorax: The muscular and bony structure of the chest.

toxicity: An undesirable result of drug use.

trachea: The main airway (windpipe) supplying both lungs.

tracheostomy: The surgical opening in the main airway, the trachea.

tracheostomy tube: The plastic, rubber, or metal tube placed into the windpipe through a surgical opening.

vaccine: An injection which may stimulate the so-called immune response which may protect an individual from a natural infection.

ventilator: The proper term for a breathing machine (Chapter VII).

virus: A group of highly contagious infectious agents that cause a variety of head colds and chest infections. Viruses are not killed by antibiotics and thus we usually have no means of preventing these and stopping the infections. Vaccination against the influenza virus is effective.

wheeze: The whistling sound of the air entering or leaving the lungs. A sign of muscular spasm of the airways and a sign of asthma.

white blood cells: The cells which generally combat infection; the white cell count is usually increased with infection.

Index